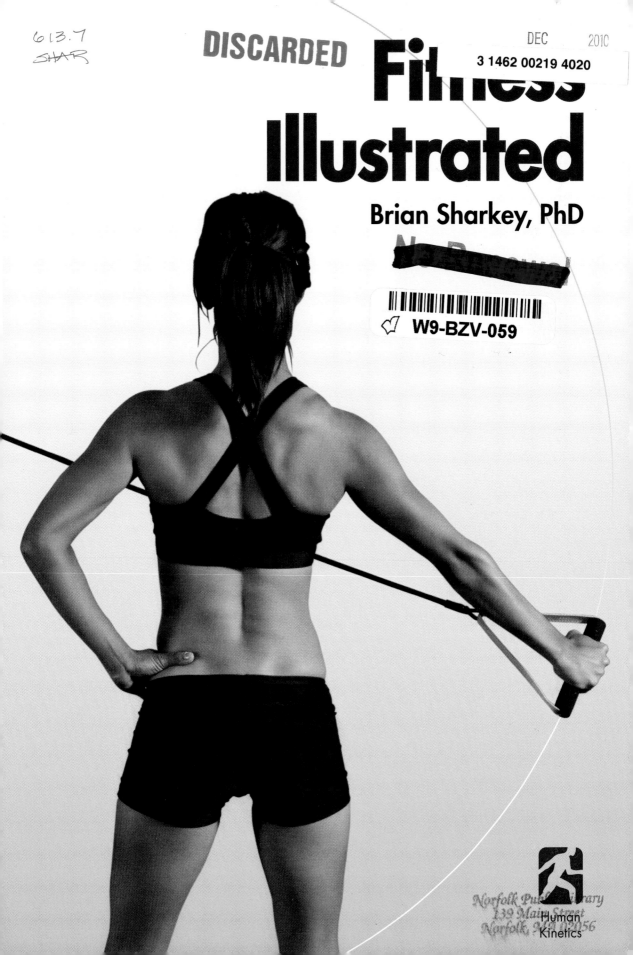

Fitness Illustrated

Brian Sharkey, PhD

Human
Kinetics

Library of Congress Cataloging-in-Publication Data

Sharkey, Brian J.
  Fitness illustrated / Brian Sharkey.
    p. cm.
  Includes bibliographical references and index.
  ISBN-13: 978-0-7360-8158-0 (soft cover)
  ISBN-10: 0-7360-8158-5 (soft cover)
  1. Physical fitness. 2. Aerobic exercises. I. Title.
  GV481.S445 2010
  613.7--dc22

                        2010003146

ISBN-10: 0-7360-8158-5 (print)
ISBN-13: 978-0-7360-8158-0 (print)

This publication is written and published to provide accurate and authoritative information relevant to the subject matter presented. It is published and sold with the understanding that the author and publisher are not engaged in rendering legal, medical, or other professional services by reason of their authorship or publication of this work. If medical or other expert assistance is required, the services of a competent professional person should be sought.

Permission notices for material reprinted in this book from other sources can be found on pages viii to xi.

The Web addresses cited in this text were current as of May 2010, unless otherwise noted.

Developmental Editor: Christine M. Drews; **Managing Editor:** Laura Podeschi; **Assistant Editor:** Dena P. Mumm; **Copyeditor:** Tom Tiller; **Indexer:** Alisha Jeddeloh; **Permission Manager:** Martha Gullo; **Graphic Designer and Graphic Artist:** Nancy Rasmus; **Cover Designer:** Keith Blomberg; **Photographer (cover):** Neil Bernstein; **Photo Asset Manager:** Laura Fitch; **Visual Production Assistant:** Joyce Brumfield; **Photo Production Manager:** Jason Allen; **Art Manager:** Kelly Hendren; **Associate Art Manager:** Alan L. Wilborn; **Art Style Development:** Joanne Brummett; **Illustrator (cover):** Jennifer Gibas, Certified Medical Illustrator, **Illustrators (interior):** Jennifer Gibas, Certified Medical Illustrator, Jessica Wheat, Medical Illustrator; **Printer:** Courier Companies, Inc.

Human Kinetics books are available at special discounts for bulk purchase. Special editions or book excerpts can also be created to specification. For details, contact the Special Sales Manager at Human Kinetics.

Printed in the United States of America   10 9 8 7 6 5 4 3 2 1

The paper in this book is certified under a sustainable forestry program.

Human Kinetics
Web site: www.HumanKinetics.com

United States: Human Kinetics
P.O. Box 5076
Champaign, IL 61825-5076
800-747-4457
e-mail: humank@hkusa.com

Canada: Human Kinetics
475 Devonshire Road Unit 100
Windsor, ON N8Y 2L5
800-465-7301 (in Canada only)
e-mail: info@hkcanada.com

Europe: Human Kinetics
107 Bradford Road
Stanningley
Leeds LS28 6AT, United Kingdom
+44 (0) 113 255 5665
e-mail: hk@hkeurope.com

Australia: Human Kinetics
57A Price Avenue
Lower Mitcham, South Australia 5062
08 8372 0999
e-mail: info@hkaustralia.com

New Zealand: Human Kinetics
P.O. Box 80
Torrens Park, South Australia 5062
0800 222 062
e-mail: info@hknewzealand.com

E4754

Ann,

You spice up my life.

Contents

Preface

I've been involved with physical activity and fitness most of my life. As a kid I was very active, until one day when my knees ached so much I was unable to walk. I was diagnosed with rheumatic fever, an acute disease characterized by fever and inflammation in the joints and the heart. During my youth I had the illness at least two times. In those days the illness required prolonged bed rest followed by a gradual return to activity. The inactivity and the disease's potential effect on the heart made me appreciate an active life. I recovered well enough to run the mile and other races in high school and college. Those experiences may explain why I decided to devote my professional life to the study of exercise and fitness.

I began college studies just as researchers were beginning to recognize the link between physical inactivity and cardiovascular disease, a topic close to my, uh, heart. Soon thereafter President Eisenhower created the President's Council on Physical Fitness to improve the fitness of military recruits. By the time I graduated from college, I knew what I wanted to do; I just didn't know where or how. Graduate studies focused that interest and prepared me for a university position involving teaching, research, and service. Since then I have devoured research journals, conducted laboratory and field studies, and published a few books. I've worked with adults, athletes, and those involved in physically demanding occupations. And I've presented papers and visited with colleagues throughout the world in an effort to better understand the benefits of physical activity and fitness. I bring this lifetime of study to the task of writing yet another fitness book.

But this book is different. It is well illustrated but not glitzy. It conveys what we know about fitness but avoids excess detail. And it allows me to clear up fallacies and misconceptions concerning exercise and its benefits. I start by answering the question *Why get fit?* You'll look at the benefits of an active life, including what you'll gain physically and psychologically. Then you'll delve into aerobic fitness—what it is, why it is important, and how you can design your own aerobic fitness program with activities that you enjoy. Next you'll look at muscular fitness, including strength, muscular endurance, and flexibility. I provide direction in creating a personalized muscular fitness program to help you reach your goals. You'll also learn what to eat for a physically active lifestyle, how you can manage your weight, and how to deal with various health issues, such as heart disease, arthritis, and fitness problems such as muscle cramps and knee pain. I explain fitness facts and fallacies so that you can be an educated fitness consumer. In the final chapter, you'll explore vitality and longevity: how you can add life to your years by becoming active now.

Whether you are just beginning or have been active for a long time, this book will pique your interest, focus your direction, and unearth the self-directed motivation that will keep you active the rest of your life.

Acknowledgments

I want to thank Rainer and Julie Martens for encouraging me to write this book, even when I doubted my ability to think visually and write sparingly. The talented staff at Human Kinetics helped bring this book to fruition. Contributors included Nancy Rasmus, graphic designer, who conceived the original design for this book and fit all the pieces together in an attractive layout; Jennifer Gibas, illustrator, who refined our sketchy illustrations; Neil Bernstein, photographer, who took the technique photos in chapter 7; Laura Podeschi, managing editor, who checked and double-checked all the details of this book; and Chris Drews, the ever-patient editor who did all she could to make the book factual and readable. To these folks and others at Human Kinetics I say thanks again for a job well done.

Credits

Figures

Page 6 (top)   Adapted, by permission, from J. Buckworth and R.K. Dishman, 2002, *Exercise psychology* (Champaign, IL: Human Kinetics), 119. Data from M. Bahrke and W.P. Morgan, 1978, "Anxiety reduction following exercise and meditation," *Cognitive Therapy and Research* 2(4): 323-333.

Page 6 (bottom)   Adapted, by permission, from J. Buckworth and R.K. Dishman, 2002, *Exercise psychology* (Champaign, IL: Human Kinetics), 140. Data from J. Fremont and L.W. Craighead, 1987, "Aerobic exercise and cognitive therapy in the treatment of dysphoric moods," *Cognitive Therapy and Research* 112: 241-251.

Page 7 (top)   Adapted, by permission, from D.L. Roth and D.S. Holmes, 1985, "Influence of physical fitness in determining the impact of stressful life events on physical and psychologic health," *Psychosomatic Medicine* 47(2): 169.

Page 7 (middle)   Adapted, by permission, from J. Buckworth and R.K. Dishman, 2002, *Exercise psychology* (Champaign, IL: Human Kinetics), 169. Data from T.M. DiLorenzo et al., 1999, "Long-term effects of aerobic exercise on psychological outcomes," *Preventive Medicine* 28(1): 75-85.

Page 7 (bottom)   Adapted, by permission, from S. Colcombe and A.F. Kramer, 2003, "Fitness effects on the cognitive function of older adults: A meta-analytic study," *Psychological Science* 14(2): 129.

Page 12   Adapted, by permission, from G.J. Balady, B. Chaitman, D. Driscoll, et al., 1998, "AHA/ACSM Joint Position Statement: Recommendations for cardiovascular screening, staffing, and emergency policies at health/fitness facilities," *Medicine & Science in Sports & Exercise* 30(6): 1009-1018.

Page 21   Adapted, by permission, from B.J. Sharkey and S.E. Gaskill, 2007, *Fitness & health*, 6th ed. (Champaign, IL: Human Kinetics), 18.

Page 26   Adapted from B.J. Sharkey and S.E. Gaskill, 2009, *Fitness and work capacity*, 2009 edition, NWCG PMS 304-2 (Boise, ID: National Wildfire Coordinating Group, Safety and Health Working Team, National Interagency Fire Center), 36.

Page 33   Adapted, by permission, from R. Martens, 2004, *Successful coaching*, 3rd ed. (Champaign, IL: Human Kinetics), 267.

Page 37   Source: Expert Panel on the Identification, Evaluation, and Treatment of Overweight in Adults, 1998, "Clinical guidelines on the identification, evaluation, and treatment of overweight and obesity in adults: Executive summary," *American Journal of Clinical Nutrition* 68(4): 899-917.

Page 217   Adapted from U.S. Department of Agriculture, 2007, *Oxygen radical absorbance capacity (ORAC) of selected foods—2007.* [Online.] Available: www.ars.usda.gov/sp2userfiles/place/12354500/data/orac/orac07.pdf [December 18, 2009].

Page 241   Reprinted, by permission, from K.E. Powell and R.S. Paffenbarger, 1985, "Workshop on epidemiologic and public health aspects of physical activity and exercise: A summary," *Public Health Reports* 100(2): 123.

Page 256   Adapted, by permission, from W.H. Ettinger, B.S. Wright, and S.N. Blair, 2006, *Fitness after 50* (Champaign: Human Kinetics), 123-124.

Page 285 (top)   Reprinted from National Center for Health Statistics, 2004, "United States life tables, 2002," *National Vital Statistics Report* 53(6): 5. [Online]. Available: http://www.cdc.gov/nchs/data/nvsr/nvsr53/nvsr53_06.pdf [February 16, 2010].

Page 285 (bottom)   Reprinted, by permission, from B.J. Sharkey and S.E. Gaskill, 2007, *Fitness & health*, 6th ed. (Champaign, IL: Human Kinetics), 349.

Page 286   Adapted, by permission, from S. Mandic, J.N. Myers, R.B. Oliveira, P. Abella, and V.F. Froelicher, 2009, "Characterizing differences in mortality at the low end of the fitness spectrum," *Medicine & Science in Sports & Exercise* 41(8): 1573-1579.

Photos

Tables

1

Activity and Fitness

Why Get Fit?

Let him that would move the world,
first move himself.

~ Socrates

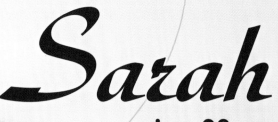

Sarah

is a 28-year-old attorney

caught up in the struggle to succeed in a high-powered urban law firm. She had been active in college but found little time for fitness in law school and now finds even less. Working more than 60 hours per week leaves her precious few hours for a personal life, let alone regular physical activity.

Her weight has crept up...

Her weight has crept up, and she lacks the vitality she enjoyed when she was active, so she wants to lose weight, regain fitness, and feel healthy again. She wants to be able to run to catch a train or plane, carry luggage through the airport without breaking a sweat, and work all day and still have the energy to go dancing. In order to meet this challenge, Sarah must set attainable goals, find time to achieve them, and get going. This book is dedicated to Sarah and to the many others who want to become active and fit, to eat right, and to experience the benefits and pleasures of an active life.

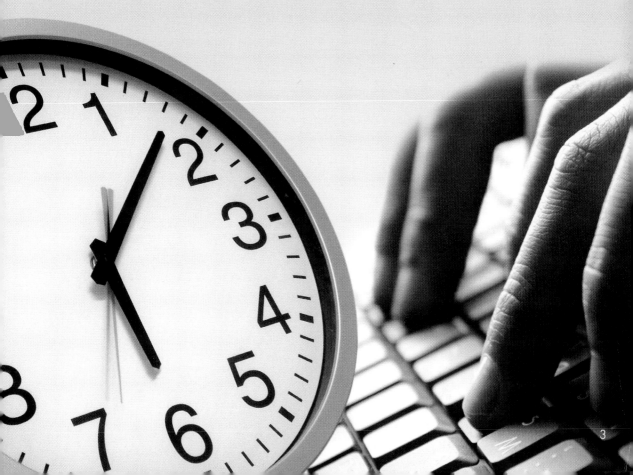

What Are the Benefits

Imagine awakening in a body that is newly transformed by several months of fitness training—a condition not unlike a state of grace, one that is inwardly sensed rather than outwardly observed. You would rise each day with the ability to carry out daily tasks with vigor and alertness, remain free of undue fatigue, enjoy your leisure pursuits, and meet unforeseen emergencies. You would have the energy and muscular fitness to carry out work and activity demands; the flexibility and balance to perform well and avoid injury; and the stamina to handle home life, work, recreation, and the inevitable unexpected demands.

If you are like many active individuals, your first thought upon waking would focus on the physical activity you planned to perform that day, as well as when and where you would do it. Indeed, when you become active and even addicted to exercise, regular physical activity becomes an indispensable part of your life. Physical activity and fitness do more than improve your performance; they also improve your physical and psychological health, thus enhancing your vigor and extending the prime of your life.

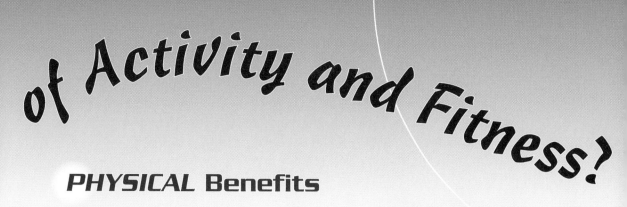

# of Activity and Fitness?

PHYSICAL Benefits

Activity and fitness . . .

Help build bone mass, reducing your chance of developing osteoporosis, osteoarthritis, and low-back pain.

Healthy, dense bone

Osteoporotic bone

Add years to your life, reduce infirmity, and extend the prime of life.

Burn calories and lower your risk of becoming overweight or developing diabetes, metabolic syndrome, and some cancers.

Belly fat can produce inflammatory molecules that enter the bloodstream, and this inflammation can lead to type 2 diabetes and heart disease. Exercise reduces belly fat and thus lowers these risks.

Reduce your risk of heart disease, hypertension, stroke, and other vascular problems.

Exercise minimizes bad, plaque-causing cholesterol and increases good, plaque-removing cholesterol.

Improve the function of your immune system.

During moderate exercise, your body increases its production of macrophages, salivary immunoglobulin A (the first defense against upper-respiratory infection), and other immune components; immune cells circulate more quickly and kill more bacteria and viruses.

Psychological Benefits

You can achieve these impressive physical benefits of activity and fitness at little or no cost while you engage in enjoyable pursuits. In turn, the benefits can dramatically reduce how much you rely on medicine and how much you spend on health care. But there are psychological benefits, too!

Activity and fitness also . . .

diminish anxiety and depression ▶

In the short term, exercise reduces anxiety in ways similar to the benefits of meditation or quiet rest. Notice the drop in anxiety from before exercise to after exercise.

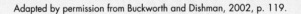

Adapted by permission from Buckworth and Dishman, 2002, p. 119.

Some studies have found that exercise is as effective as psychotherapy in reducing depressive symptoms. Notice the decrease in symptoms of depression from the start of treatment to week 18. The exercise in this study was running.

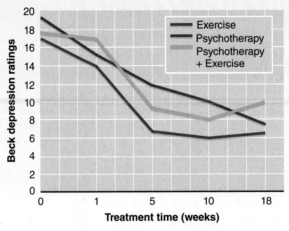

Adapted by permission from Buckworth and Dishman, 2002, p. 140.

control stress and minimize its negative effects on the body

A high level of stress can be associated with poorer physical health, especially for people with a low fitness level. Life stress has less impact on the physical health of fit people.

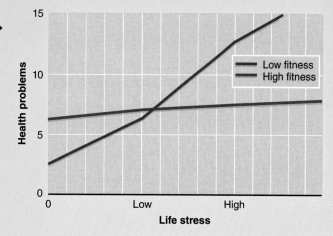

Adapted by permission from Roth and Holmes, 1985, p. 169.

improve self-esteem
(how you feel about yourself)

self-concept
(what you think about yourself)

and body image

Self-esteem regarding one's body increased after 12 weeks of cycling 4 times per week for 30 minutes each session.

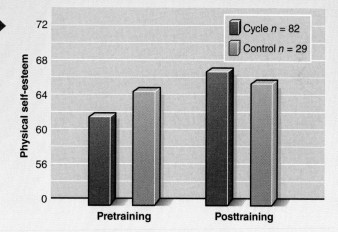

Adapted by permission from Buckworth and Dishman, 2002, p. 169.

improve cognition and problem solving

This shows the effects of fitness training on four different brain tasks. The purple bars illustrate the cognitive functioning of people who did not exercise. The red bars illustrate the cognitive functioning of people who were part of an aerobic fitness training group. Exercise really does help your brain!

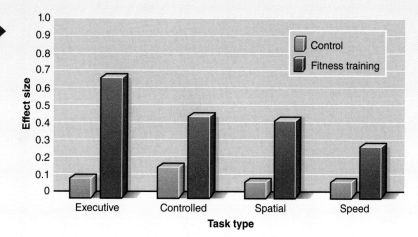

Executive = planning of mental procedures; Controlled = requiring cognitive control; Spatial = remembering visual information; Speed = low-level neurological planning (e.g., simple reaction time).

Adapted by permission from Colcombe and Kramer, 2003, p. 129.

Psychological Benefits

Activity and fitness also . . .

help you sleep better, if activity is performed well before bedtime ▶

▶ add life to your years
(activity and fitness improve interest in and enjoyment of intimacy!)

Our bodies were designed to move—not to sit in front of a desk, computer, video game, or television set. Physical activity and fitness work (or training) focus your movement and ensure that you will achieve the impressive list of benefits just discussed. They also improve your posture, muscle tone, and appearance. Some people even report a spiritual dimension of experience associated with fitness.

FitFact

You'll be healthier and feel better emotionally once you become physically active.

How Much Do You Need?

In 1995, the American College of Sports Medicine and the Centers for Disease Control recommended that every adult should engage in 30 minutes of moderate activity on most days of the week. In 2002, in light of the national epidemic of overweight and obesity, the Institute of Medicine recommended 1 hour of daily activity to achieve greater health benefits and to maintain healthy body weight. What are the latest recommendations?

♥ *Physical Activity Guidelines*

You can enjoy the substantial health benefits available from physical activity by following the *2008 Physical Activity Guidelines for Americans*, published by the U.S. Department of Health and Human Services.

- Adults should do 2 hours and 30 minutes a week of moderate-intensity—or 1 hour and 15 minutes (75 minutes) a week of vigorous-intensity—aerobic physical activity, or an equivalent combination of moderate- and vigorous-intensity aerobic physical activity. Aerobic activity should be performed in episodes of at least 10 minutes, preferably spread throughout the week.

> If you are active for a little over 20 minutes a day, every day of the week, or for 30 minutes on 5 days a week, you meet this recommendation.

- You can gain added health benefits by increasing to 5 hours (300 min) a week of moderate-intensity aerobic physical activity, or 2 hours and 30 minutes a week of vigorous-intensity physical activity, or an equivalent combination of both.

> You can meet this mark by performing 1 hour of moderate-intensity exercise on 5 days a week.

- Adults should also perform muscle-strengthening activities that involve all major muscle groups on 2 or more days per week.

If this sounds like too much for you, don't worry. We'll show you how to start small and finish strong.

What Are Physical Activity and Fitness?

Physical Activity

I talk about physical activity because the term *exercise* carries a negative connotation for some. *Exercise* suggests a requirement, whereas the term *physical activity* suggests something you choose to do. You might choose from a variety of enjoyable pursuits, including walking, gardening, sports, and recreational activities. Doing regular physical activity will improve your health and reduce your risk of many health problems, including heart disease, which is the number one killer of men and women in many industrialized nations. Exactly how does physical activity lead to improved fitness and other health benefits? Read on.

Fitness

The term *fitness* includes two main categories: aerobic fitness and muscular fitness. **Aerobic fitness** refers to your ability to carry out continuous tasks, such as walking, running, cycling, cross-country skiing, paddling, and other large-muscle activities. When you engage in an activity such as walking or jogging at a level above your normal daily level (or load), you overload your muscles and their support systems, including your heart and lungs. If you repeat the exercise regularly (e.g., every other day), your body begins to adapt to the overload imposed

OVER

by the exercise, and we call these many adaptations the *training effect*. The exercise signals genes in your muscle fibers and support systems to initiate changes that enable more exercise in the future. As you improve your aerobic fitness, you enhance your ability to burn fat and manage your body weight even as you reduce your risk for heart disease, diabetes, and some cancers.

Muscular fitness includes strength, muscle endurance, and flexibility, as well as power (strength exerted as fast as possible). You need muscular fitness in order to carry out daily tasks and meet unforeseen emergencies. In addition, as you age, you need muscular fitness to do simple things such as get out of a chair, climb stairs, or open a jar—in other words, to remain independent.

Muscular and aerobic fitness depend on the old adage *use it or lose it.* If you allow your muscular fitness to decline, your life becomes more difficult. If you maintain it, you have the capacity to live a full, active, independent life. Of course, fitness training improves the function of your heart, but when your heart is working well, oxygen and nutrients reach your muscles, and that is where the major changes take place.

In chapters 2 through 4, I will help you make a plan for aerobic fitness, and in chapters 5 to 7, you'll learn how to create a muscular fitness program. Before we proceed, however, we must consider some of the risks of exertion.

Skeletal muscle, not the heart, is the primary target of aerobic and muscular fitness training.

Recycle. Do Something Good For The Earth

load

Health Screen

Assess your health needs by marking all *true* statements.

History

You have had:

__ a heart attack
__ heart surgery
__ cardiac catheterization
__ coronary angioplasty (PTCA)
__ pacemaker/implantable cardiac defibrillator/rhythm disturbance
__ heart valve disease
__ heart failure
__ heart transplantation
__ congenital heart disease

If you marked any of the statements in this section, consult your health care provider before engaging in exercise. You may need to use a facility that offers a medically qualified staff.

Symptoms

__ You experience chest discomfort with exertion.
__ You experience unreasonable breathlessness.
__ You experience dizziness, fainting, or blackouts.
__ You take heart medications.

Other Health Issues

__ You have musculoskeletal problems.
__ You have concerns about the safety of exercise.
__ You take prescription medication(s).
__ You are pregnant.

Cardiovascular Risk Factors

__ You are a man older than 45 years.
__ You are a woman older than 55 years or you have had a hysterectomy or you are postmenopausal.
__ You smoke.
__ Your blood pressure is greater than 140/90.
__ You don't know your blood pressure.
__ You take blood pressure medication.
__ Your blood cholesterol level is greater than 240 mg/dl.
__ You don't know your blood cholesterol level.
__ You have a close blood relative who had a heart attack before age 55 (father or brother) or before age 65 (mother or sister).
__ You have diabetes or take medicine to control your blood sugar.
__ You are physically inactive (i.e., you do not get at least 30 minutes of physical activity on at least 3 days per week).
__ You are more than 20 pounds (9 kg) overweight. (You can use the BMI chart on p. 37 to find out.)

If you marked two or more of the statements in this section, you should consult your health care provider before engaging in exercise. You might benefit from using a facility that offers a professionally qualified exercise staff to guide your exercise program.

__ None of the above is true.

You should be able to exercise safely without consulting your health care provider in almost any facility that meets your exercise program needs.

Adapted by permission from Balady, Chaitman, and Driscoll, 1998.

Risks of Exertion

Is exercise safe? Exertion is associated with just 10 percent of all heart attacks, meaning that 90 percent of all heart attacks occur at rest (Thompson et al. 2007). At the same time, the American Heart Association has identified physical *in*activity (along with hypertension, elevated cholesterol, and smoking) as a major risk factor for heart disease.

If you are inactive, you are *50 times* more likely to experience heart problems during exertion than those who are active (Siscovick, LaPorte, and Newman 1985). Thus, if you have been inactive, you must become physically active *before* you engage in fitness training. By *training*, I mean deliberately increasing your level of activity for the purpose of becoming fit. To become physically active, start a 4- to 6-week walking program, slowly increasing distance and pace until you can walk 2 to 3 miles (about 3 to 5 km) at a good pace. If you are older or have been sedentary for a long time, you may need to walk for more than 6 weeks before you begin fitness training.

To ensure that you are ready for vigorous activity and training, complete the AHA/ACSM Health/Fitness Facility Preparticipation Screening Questionnaire recommended by the American Heart Association and the American College of Sports Medicine. I've called it a Health Screen, and you can find it on the previous page.

Keys to Activity and Fitness

➤ Fitness offers abundant benefits. From a healthy heart to a healthy outlook on life, being physically active boosts your physical and psychological well-being.

➤ Adults should do 2 hours and 30 minutes a week of moderate-intensity physical activity.

➤ You become fit by challenging your body to do more than it is used to doing.

➤ Become physically active before you engage in fitness training.

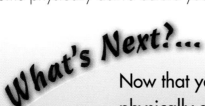

What's Next?...

Now that you know the benefits of being physically active, check out chapter 2 to discover how your body will change as you become aerobically fit.

2

Understanding Aerobic Fitness

O$_2$ and You

Fitness can neither be
bought nor bestowed.
Like honor, it must
be earned.

~ Anonymous

Ed

was a Postal Service employee

who managed to maintain his fitness while walking his route in hilly Seattle. After retirement, he tried several forms of activity before settling on the bicycle as a way to maintain fitness. He joined a local riding group to increase his capacity. In time, he was doing longer rides, including his first century (100 miles [about 160 km]). Then he became interested in bicycle touring and began doing extended rides during which he carried food, clothing, and a tent and sleeping bag.

He loved the rhythm of the ride...

He loved the rhythm of the ride: Get up early for breakfast, break camp, and ride until lunch; then ride several more hours, stop to set up camp, eat dinner, socialize, and head off to his sleeping bag. He started reading a cycling magazine, and that is where he learned of an epic bicycle adventure. At the age of 64, Ed joined a much younger group for a ride from Anchorage to Fairbanks, Alaska, and then south to Long Beach, California—a distance of 4,400 miles (nearly 7,100 km), including 500 miles (about 800 km) on gravel roads. The group completed the ride in 3 months, averaging about 50 miles (80 km) a day, and—despite a fall, bruised ribs, and other minor discomforts— Ed was right there with the young folks. As they approached the end, Ed began to think about his next aerobic adventure.

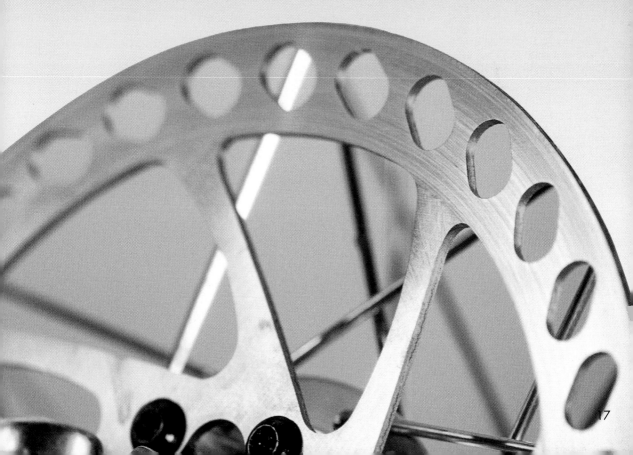

Why Do Aerobic

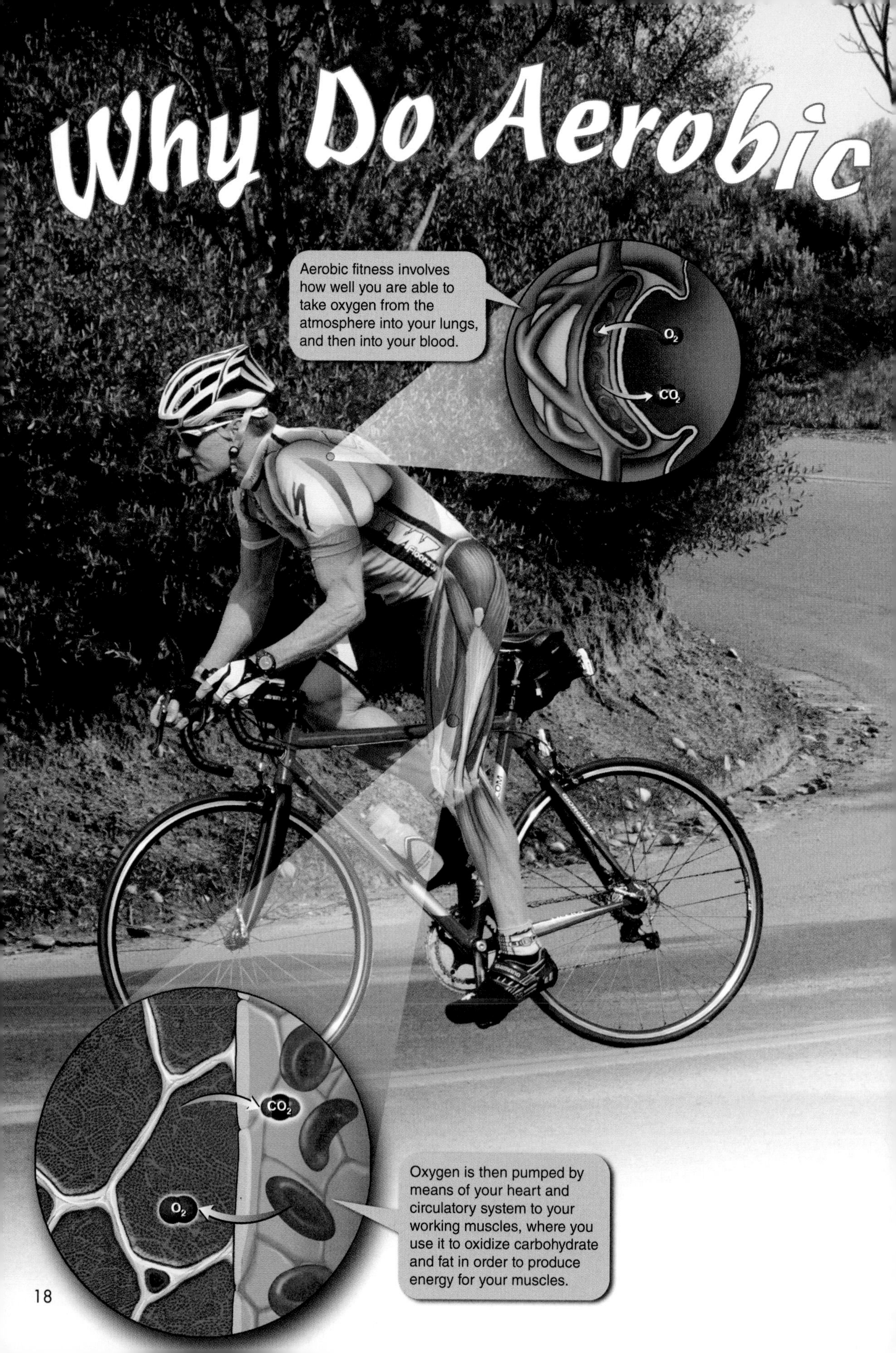

Aerobic fitness involves how well you are able to take oxygen from the atmosphere into your lungs, and then into your blood.

O_2

CO_2

CO_2

O_2

Oxygen is then pumped by means of your heart and circulatory system to your working muscles, where you use it to oxidize carbohydrate and fat in order to produce energy for your muscles.

Exercise?

Somewhere above the pace of your normal daily activities, but well below maximal effort, you will find aerobic exercise. If you do aerobic exercise often enough, you will improve your aerobic fitness, and as your fitness improves, you'll enhance your health, appearance, vitality, and quality of life.

The respiratory and circulatory systems are important in aerobic exercise—they supply oxygen and nutrients—but it is the skeletal muscles that produce movement. The most important benefits of aerobic exercise occur within the muscles themselves. Perhaps the greatest advantage of aerobic fitness is that it improves your ability to burn fat as a source of energy.

FitFact

Aerobic fitness describes the health and capacity of your lungs, heart, circulatory system, and, most important, skeletal muscles.

Aerobic exercises include rhythmic, large-muscle activities such as brisk walking, jogging, cycling, swimming, cross-country skiing, and rowing.

➤ Such activities make your lungs, heart, and muscles do sustained work at an elevated level and thus cause those systems to adapt to the increase in workload.

➤ Aerobic exercise can improve your health and help you live longer; regular aerobic exercise improves your aerobic fitness, and improved fitness enhances your health.

➤ As you become aerobically fit, your quality of life may improve physically, psychologically, and socially.

➤ Aerobic fitness enhances your appearance, boosts your self-confidence and body image, and opens the door to a challenging new world filled with compelling experiences and engaging people.

The more you exercise, the less chance you have of heart disease.

With improved aerobic fitness, you will be able to run to catch the bus or taxi, walk briskly through an airport without becoming breathless, keep up with the kids or grandkids, and dance the night away with your significant other.

Aerobic fitness is synonymous with endurance or stamina. It describes the ability, partially inherited and partially trained, to engage in prolonged endeavors. Those who pursue fitness earn far more than enhanced health and performance. For many, the process becomes more important than the goal, providing discipline, challenge, and time for reflection.

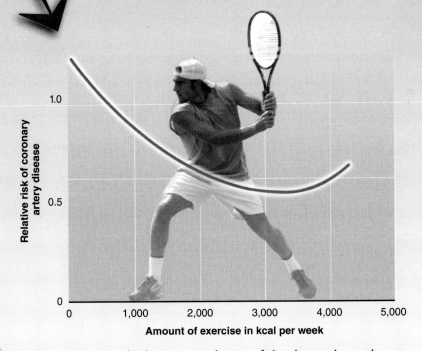

The more you exercise, the lower your chance of developing heart disease.

We think the increase on the right-hand side of the graph results from the small number of cases that report burning more than 3,500 calories per week.

Adapted by permission from Sharkey and Gaskill, 2007, p. 18.

Don't Call It Cardio!

Back in the 1950s, our knowledge of fitness was limited to the effect of training on the heart. Training led to a reduction in the resting and exercise heart rates, so it was called cardiovascular fitness. As we began to understand the effect of training on oxygen intake and oxygen transport, it came to be called cardiorespiratory fitness. Then, in 1967, Dr. John Holloszy published a landmark study of the effects of training on skeletal muscle fibers (i.e., the cells found inside such muscles as your biceps, quadriceps, and hamstrings). The study showed that training doubled oxidative enzymes and the trained muscle's ability to use oxygen. In other words, the more a person trains, the better his or her muscles use oxygen. From that point onward, we have defined fitness as a person's maximal ability to take in, transport, and use oxygen.

The term *cardio* does describe one part of aerobic fitness, but it ignores the important effects of training on muscle fibers. Once you understand the full picture, you can design your fitness training program the right way. You can't become aerobically fit simply by raising your heart rate; if you could, then the mere elevation of heart rate from receiving a scare would improve fitness. Nor can you become fit by using any old variety of muscles to simply raise heart rate. Instead, you need to systematically use your large muscle groups in order to get oxygen circulating to the muscles used in the activity (running, cycling, etc.). Heart rate is sometimes used as a measure of how much oxygen you are using in order to gauge exercise intensity. But skeletal muscle (in the muscles used in the activity) is the target of training. The role of your heart is to supply the working muscles with oxygen and energy.

Aerobic Metabolism

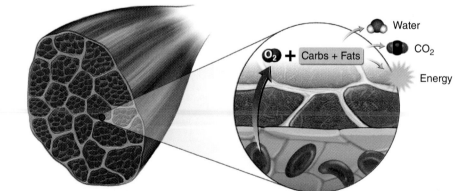

Inside your muscles, a chemical reaction occurs between oxygen and fat or carbohydrate. This reaction is called oxidation. When oxidation occurs within a muscle cell, carbohydrate and fat from food react chemically with oxygen, and energy is released in such a way that it can be converted to movement by your muscles. This chemical reaction also produces carbon dioxide and water, which are removed from your body through breathing and sweating. This entire process is also called aerobic metabolism. When the muscle can't get enough oxygen, much less energy is produced.

Aerobic fitness
is the ability to

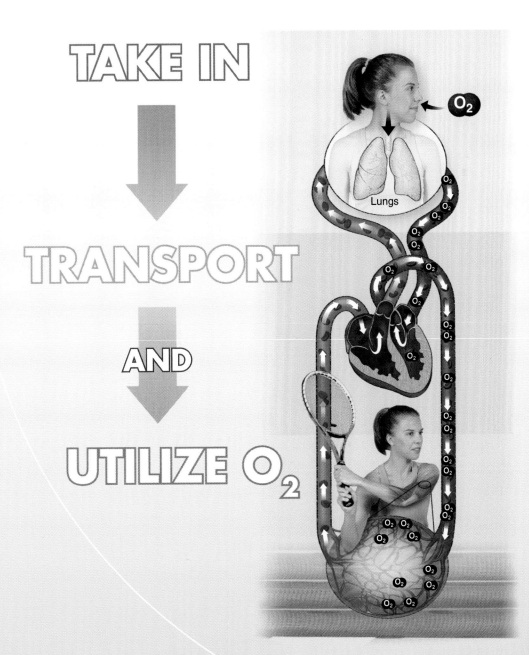

TAKE IN

TRANSPORT

AND

UTILIZE O_2

Measuring Aerobic Fitness

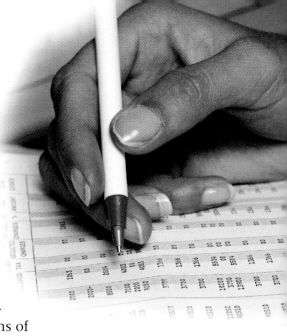

Before you start a program of physical activity, you might want to measure your aerobic fitness. That way, once you have been active for a while, you will be able to gauge how much your aerobic fitness has improved. Aerobic fitness is usually measured by means of a treadmill or bicycle test. The person being tested is fitted with ECG electrodes and a breathing valve to direct exhaled air to a computer that measures oxygen intake. After a warm-up, the person exercises by taking on increasing workloads until he or she cannot continue. The highest level of oxygen intake is referred to either as the maximal oxygen intake ($\dot{V}O_2$max) or as aerobic fitness (usually reported in milliliters of oxygen per kilogram of body weight per minute [mlO_2/kg/min]). Since maximal oxygen intake is related to body weight, weight loss can improve aerobic fitness since you divide the $\dot{V}O_2$max by body weight.

Tests You Can Use

Since you probably don't keep electrodes around your home, you can estimate your aerobic fitness by using an activity index or a running test.

Activity Index

You can gauge your current level of activity by using the activity index presented on the following page. It illustrates how increasing the intensity, duration, and frequency of your exercise can improve your fitness. Just circle the scores that match your typical activity level, multiply the numbers as indicated, and use the key at the bottom to see where you rate. If your score is below 40, you should begin—today—to increase your daily activity.

Activity Index

Based on your regular daily activity, calculate your activity index by multiplying your score for each category (score = intensity × duration × frequency).

	Score	Daily activity
Intensity	5	Sustained effort with heavy breathing and perspiration
	4	Intermittent heavy breathing and perspiration (e.g., tennis, racquetball)
	3	Moderately heavy (e.g., recreational jogging, cycling)
	2	Moderate (e.g., walking, volleyball, softball)
	1	Light (e.g., fishing, gardening)
Duration	4	More than 60 minutes
	3	30 to 60 minutes
	2	20 to 29 minutes
	1	Fewer than 20 minutes
Frequency	5	Daily or almost daily
	4	3 to 5 times a week
	3	1 or 2 times a week
	2	A few times a month
	1	Less often than once a month

Evaluation and Fitness Category

Score	Evaluation	Fitness category*
100	Very active lifestyle	High
80 to 99	Active and healthy	Very good
60 to 79	Active	Good
40 to 59	Acceptable (could be better)	Fair
20 to 39	Not good enough	Poor
Under 20	Sedentary	Very poor

*Index score is associated with aerobic fitness.

Adapted from Kasari, 1976, p. 46.

RUNNING

Run Test

If you are a runner, you can estimate your aerobic fitness by means of a run test. The 1.5-mile (2.4 km) run assesses aerobic fitness for runners. If you're not a runner, use the walk–jog test found in chapter 4.

Here's how to do the 1.5-mile (2.4 km) run test:

1 Mark out a 1.5-mile (2.4 km) course. Make sure the route is flat so that you get a fair time.

2 Jog or run the course as fast as you can and record your time in minutes and seconds.

3 Use the chart below to evaluate your result:

➤ Subtract the altitude adjustment from your run time.

➤ Use the graph to find your score.

If you are running, you can do this test every 6 weeks to see how you are progressing in your aerobic fitness training. If you are cycling, use a bicycle.

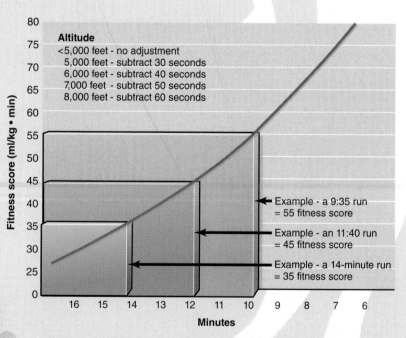

Altitude
<5,000 feet - no adjustment
5,000 feet - subtract 30 seconds
6,000 feet - subtract 40 seconds
7,000 feet - subtract 50 seconds
8,000 feet - subtract 60 seconds

Example - a 9:35 run = 55 fitness score

Example - an 11:40 run = 45 fitness score

Example - a 14-minute run = 35 fitness score

The 1.5-mile (2.4 km) run test. Subtract altitude adjustment from your run time, and then use the graph to find your score.

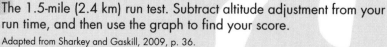
Adapted from Sharkey and Gaskill, 2009, p. 36.

Specificity of Exercise

The Effects of Exercise Training Are Specific

When you train, the muscles you use change and adapt. Since training is specific, it is important that you decide what you are training for.

➤ If you intend to run a 10K race, train by running.

➤ If you want to be fit for an upcoming canoe outing, train by paddling.

➤ Whatever you intend to do—a long hike, a swim, or a bicycle trip—train appropriately. Focus your training on the activity you intend to improve. Don't assume your fitness in one activity will completely transfer to being fit to perform in another activity.

It works the same way with testing: Since the effects of training are specific, testing must also be specific. If you're a runner, don't test yourself on a bicycle; if you're a cyclist, don't test yourself on a treadmill. You can read more about specificity in chapters 3 and 5.

FitFact

Training is specific. Running will help you run better. Swimming will help you swim better. Know what you are training for, and then train and test with that same activity.

To get better at an activity, you have to train with that same activity.

Effects of Aerobic Endurance Training

Aerobic endurance training is good for your health and performance. Let's look at the effects of training on your respiratory and circulatory systems and on the muscles, which are the target of training.

Supply and Support Systems

Aerobic means in the presence of oxygen, which is the key to physical activity and fitness. Oxygen utilization in trained muscles is what gives you the stamina to be active for long periods of time. Let's consider how air gets into your lungs and how the circulation of your blood carries oxygen and energy to your working muscles.

Respiration

People often say "I ran out of wind" or "I couldn't catch my breath." The sense of fatigue associated with breathlessness during exercise is linked to the major functions of respiration—getting oxygen into the lungs and getting rid of carbon dioxide.

RESPIRATION

Air is made up of about 21 percent oxygen. Air enters the lungs when your diaphragm and other respiratory muscles contract and create an area of lower pressure.

O_2

O_2

Inhale

Exhale

The average lung holds 2 to 5 liters of air.

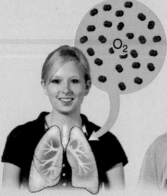

Trained individuals take bigger breaths, thus requiring fewer breaths to get the same amount of oxygen.

Untrained individuals take shallow breaths and thus need more breaths to get sufficient oxygen.

Before training, you might inhale 2 liters of air per breath; after training, you might inhale 3 liters per breath. Thus, if you need 60 liters of air per minute, your breathing rate would decrease from 30 to 20 breaths per minute.

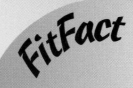
Before training

60 liters/min = 30 breaths × 2 liters per breath

After training

60 liters/min = 20 breaths × 3 liters per breath

This means that your respiratory muscles wouldn't have to work as hard to take in the same amount of oxygen. Training makes respiration more efficient, putting more oxygen into your lungs, where it can find its way into your bloodstream. As a result, more oxygen will reach your muscles!

Circulation

Your circulatory system consists of your heart, blood, and blood vessels. Once you take a breath, oxygen hooks a ride on the hemoglobin in your

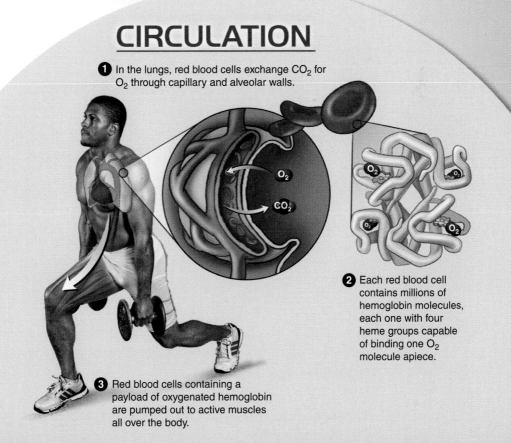

CIRCULATION

❶ In the lungs, red blood cells exchange CO_2 for O_2 through capillary and alveolar walls.

O_2

CO_2

❷ Each red blood cell contains millions of hemoglobin molecules, each one with four heme groups capable of binding one O_2 molecule apiece.

❸ Red blood cells containing a payload of oxygenated hemoglobin are pumped out to active muscles all over the body.

red blood cells and is carried to your working muscles via your blood vessels. The blood volume in an adult human body averages about 5 liters, and one result of training is an increase of 10 to 15 percent in blood volume—a major benefit that I will discuss in a moment.

Your heart is the ultimate endurance muscle, beating about 70 times per minute (when you are at rest) every minute of your life. Aerobic endurance training brings about subtle changes in your heart, and more dramatic changes take place during prolonged periods of serious training. Two obvious effects of training are a lower resting heart rate and a lower exercise heart rate.

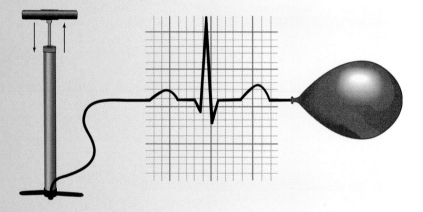

Cardiac output = heart rate × stroke volume

The amount of blood pumped by the heart (cardiac output) = heart rate × the volume of blood pumped per stroke (stroke volume)

For example, following a period of training (e.g., 6 weeks), your heart rate while jogging might drop from 150 beats per minute (bpm) to 125 bpm. Heart rate declines because stroke volume increases. What causes this rise in stroke volume and the corresponding drop in heart rate? At least half of the effect is due to the increase in blood volume that occurs with training. Your heart is a pump: Put more blood in the chamber, and more is pumped out. If your blood volume goes from 5 to 5.5 or 5.75 liters, your heart becomes more efficient, leading to lower resting and exercise heart rates.

Typical aerobic endurance training leads to subtle changes in heart function. Intense or long-term training done by endurance athletes can influence the size (diameter) of your heart muscle fibers, the volume of your heart chambers, and the thickness of your heart chamber walls. Training also increases the capillary density around your muscles in order to improve oxygen delivery.

Your performance improves with training because your respiration and circulation become more efficient and thus deliver oxygen more effectively to your working muscles. Your health improves because training

➤ reduces your blood pressure,
➤ improves your arterial elasticity,
➤ enhances blood flow in your coronary arteries in the heart,
➤ burns fat, and
➤ lowers cholesterol and triglycerides in your blood.

So, as you improve your fitness, you'll feel better because your heart is not working as hard, you'll be able to do activity more easily, and you'll enjoy some great health benefits!

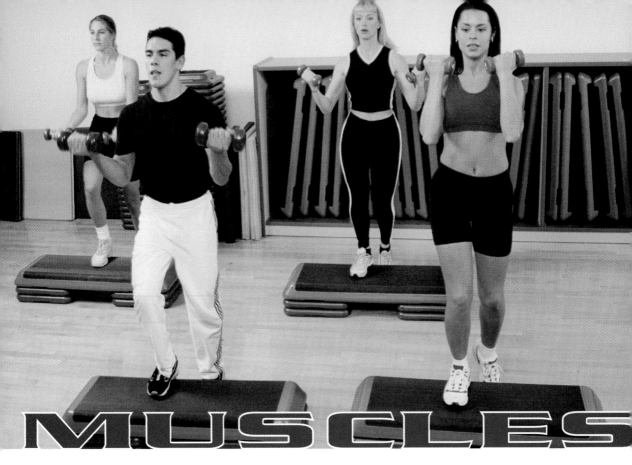

MUSCLES

Muscles

The targets of your training are the muscles used in the activity (e.g., running). Each of your muscles contains thousands of spaghetti-like fibers, which in turn contain proteins that cause your muscles to shorten and produce movement and force. Muscle fibers contract in groups when stimulated by their motor nerve, which is made up of many motor neurons. Aerobic endurance training improves the delivery of oxygen to your muscles, improves the energy pathways that burn fat and carbohydrate, and improves your use of fat as fuel for energy to power your muscle contractions. In other words, aerobic training is good for your muscles and your health.

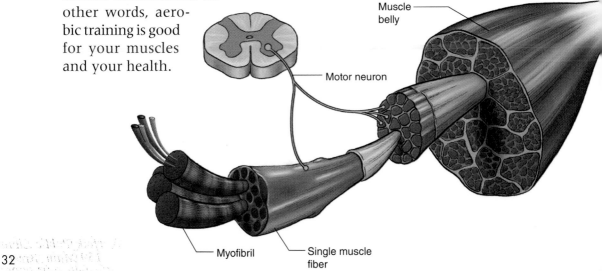

Muscle belly

Motor neuron

Myofibril

Single muscle fiber

ENERGY

Energy

Energy—the ability to do work—comes from the sun, is converted into chemical compounds by plants and animals, and eventually finds its way into your body in the form of carbohydrate, fat, and protein molecules. Chemical breakdown of these molecules through the process of oxidation releases stored energy and uses it to power the human machine. Carbohydrate and fat provide most of the energy for your muscles; protein provides a small percentage, except when energy intake is limited, as in food restriction or starvation. In those cases, the body calls on its protein stores to provide most of the energy. This can have an adverse effect on muscle and other tissue. But for most physical activity in typical situations, carbohydrate and fat provide energy for muscle contractions.

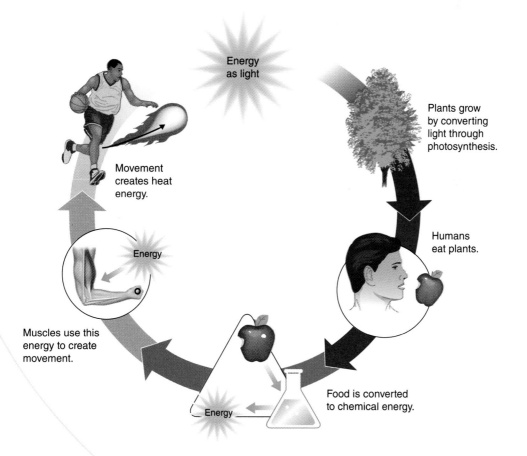

Energy as light

Plants grow by converting light through photosynthesis.

Humans eat plants.

Food is converted to chemical energy.

Energy

Muscles use this energy to create movement.

Energy

Movement creates heat energy.

Adapted by permission from Martens, 2004, p. 267.

ENERGY

Sources of Energy for Different Levels of Activity

Intensity	Activity examples	Source of energy
Light	Leisure walking Light housework Chopping vegetables Mowing the lawn with a riding mower Playing catch	**Mainly fat** Primarily from fat carried in blood with only a little expen- diture from muscle triglyceride

Moderate	Brisk walking
	Recreational jogging
	Bicycling at a slow pace
	  (10 miles [16 km] per hour)
	Paddling in a pool
	Light weightlifting
	Vigorous vacuuming
	Tai chi, yoga, Pilates
	  (though sometimes these
	  are light intensity)
	Golfing without a cart
	Mowing the lawn with a
	  power mower
		Fat and carbohydrate
		Primarily from blood-
		borne–free fatty acids,
		muscle triglyceride, and
		carbohydrate stored in muscle
		(glycogen)

High-intensity
endurance
exercise
	Long-distance running
	Bicycling at a medium pace
	  (13 miles [21 km] per hour)
	Doubles tennis
	Swimming laps
	Stair climbing
	Vigorous yardwork (digging
	  in the garden, hauling
	  material in a wheelbarrow)
	High-intensity aerobic dance
		**Mainly carbohydrate with
		some contribution from fat**
		Primarily muscle glycogen
		with some blood glucose

High-intensity
sprint-like
exercise
	50-meter dash
	Running to catch the bus,
	  taxi, or train
	Running to the next base
	  in softball
	Chopping wood in short
	  bursts
	Weightlifting with vigorous
	  effort
		Mainly carbohydrate
		Primarily muscle glycogen

Protein is also a source of energy for most activities, but it contributes only a very small percentage at all intensities.

Fat is used to power light and moderate activity; as exercise intensity increases, carbohydrate use rises and fat use falls. While most of us have enough carbohydrate to fuel about 80 minutes of effort, we store enough fat to fuel several hundred miles of running. Small amounts of carbohydrate are stored in the liver and muscles. Large amounts of fat are stored in adipose tissue (fat storage areas located around the body).

FitFact

Aerobic fitness improves your muscles' ability to use fat, and thus contributes to weight loss and improvements in your health and performance.

Effects of Training on Muscles

When you train, you not only improve your respiration and circulation but also benefit your muscles in important ways. Muscle cells include certain parts called mitochondria, which are cellular powerhouses. Mitochondria are the site of a chemical process in which oxygen is used to make energy from carbohydrate and fat. When you train, you increase the volume of your muscle mitochondria, which means that your muscles can burn more carbohydrate and fat. Training also doubles your muscles' ability to use oxygen, so endurance-trained muscles are better able to use fat as an energy source. So if you want to burn fat, train for endurance!

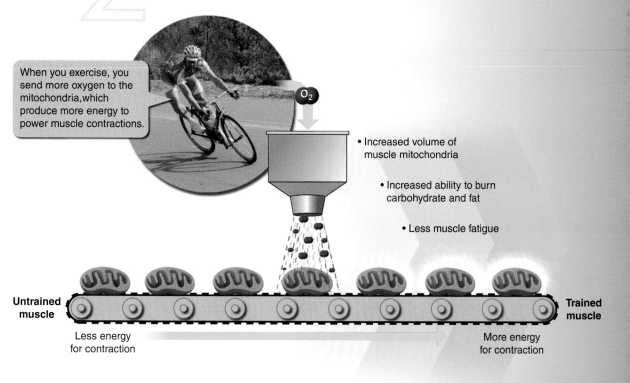

When you exercise, you send more oxygen to the mitochondria, which produce more energy to power muscle contractions.

O_2

• Increased volume of muscle mitochondria

• Increased ability to burn carbohydrate and fat

• Less muscle fatigue

Untrained muscle

Trained muscle

Less energy for contraction

More energy for contraction

Body Fat

Aerobic endurance training has a profound effect on body fat. On average, young males have 15 to 20 percent fat and young females have 20 to 30 percent fat. Use your height and weight and the body mass index (BMI) chart on the following page to determine whether you have excess body fat. BMI values above 25 are considered overweight, and those above 30 are considered obese. With training and improved fitness, your percent body fat declines, along with your weight. Aerobic endurance training burns fat and lowers your BMI score.

Fat is stored in adipose tissue, which is located beneath the skin and around the organs. Fat is the preferred fuel during moderate physical activity.

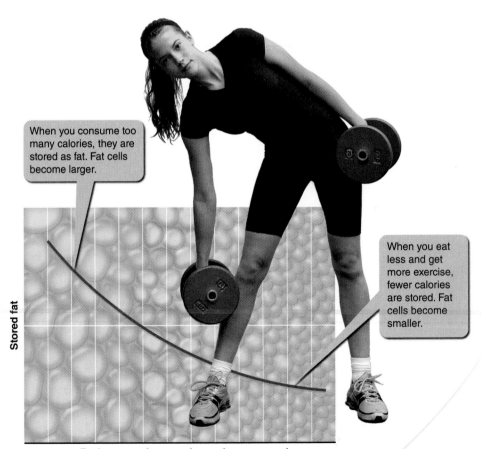

When you consume too many calories, they are stored as fat. Fat cells become larger.

When you eat less and get more exercise, fewer calories are stored. Fat cells become smaller.

Stored fat

Eat less, exercise more (expend more energy)

Height (in) / Weight (lb)	49	51	53	55	57	59	61	63	65	67	69	71	73	75	77	79	81	83
66	19	18	16	15	14	13	12	12	11	10	10	9	9	8	8	8	7	7
70	20	19	18	16	15	14	13	13	12	11	10	10	9	9	8	8	8	7
75	22	20	19	17	16	15	14	13	12	12	11	10	10	9	9	9	8	8
79	23	21	20	18	17	16	15	14	13	12	12	11	11	10	9	9	9	8
84	24	22	21	19	18	17	16	15	14	13	12	12	11	11	10	10	9	9
88	26	24	22	20	19	18	17	16	15	14	13	12	12	11	11	10	10	9
92	27	25	23	21	20	19	17	16	15	15	14	13	12	12	11	11	10	10
97	28	26	24	22	21	20	18	17	16	15	14	14	13	12	12	11	10	10
101	29	27	25	23	22	20	19	18	17	16	15	14	13	13	12	12	11	10
106	31	28	26	24	23	21	20	19	18	17	16	15	14	13	13	12	11	11
110	32	30	27	26	24	22	21	20	18	17	16	15	15	14	13	13	11	11
114	33	31	29	27	25	23	22	20	19	18	17	16	15	14	14	13	12	12
119	35	32	30	28	26	24	22	21	20	19	18	17	16	15	14	14	13	12
123	36	33	31	29	27	25	23	22	21	19	18	17	16	16	15	14	13	13
128	37	34	32	30	28	26	24	23	21	20	19	18	17	16	15	15	14	13
132	38	36	33	31	29	27	25	23	22	21	20	19	18	17	16	15	14	14
136	40	37	34	32	29	28	26	24	23	21	20	19	18	17	16	16	15	14
141	41	38	35	33	30	28	27	25	24	22	21	20	19	18	17	16	15	15
145	42	39	36	34	31	29	27	26	24	23	22	20	19	18	17	17	16	15
150	44	40	37	35	32	30	28	27	25	24	22	21	20	19	18	17	16	15
154	45	41	38	36	33	31	29	27	26	24	23	22	20	19	18	18	17	16
158	46	43	40	37	34	32	30	28	26	25	24	22	21	20	19	18	17	16
163	47	44	41	38	35	33	31	29	27	26	24	23	22	20	19	19	18	17
167	49	45	42	39	36	34	32	30	28	26	25	23	22	21	20	19	18	17
172	50	46	43	40	37	35	32	30	29	27	25	24	23	22	21	20	19	18
176	51	47	44	41	38	36	33	31	29	28	26	25	23	22	21	20	19	18
180	52	49	45	42	39	36	34	32	30	28	27	25	24	23	22	21	20	19
185	54	50	46	43	40	37	35	33	31	29	27	26	25	23	22	21	20	19
189	55	51	47	44	41	38	36	34	32	30	28	27	25	24	23	22	20	20
194	56	52	48	45	42	39	37	34	32	30	29	27	26	24	23	22	21	20
198	58	53	49	46	43	40	37	35	33	31	29	28	26	25	24	23	21	20
202	59	54	50	47	44	41	38	36	34	32	30	28	27	25	24	23	22	21
207	60	56	52	48	45	42	39	37	35	33	31	29	27	26	25	24	22	21
211	61	57	53	49	46	43	40	38	35	33	31	30	28	27	25	24	23	22
216	63	58	54	50	47	44	41	38	36	34	32	30	29	27	26	25	23	22
220	64	59	55	51	48	44	42	39	37	35	33	31	29	28	26	25	24	23
224	65	60	56	52	49	45	42	40	37	35	33	31	30	28	27	26	24	23
229	67	62	57	53	49	46	43	41	38	36	34	32	30	29	27	26	25	24
233	68	63	58	54	50	47	44	41	39	37	35	33	31	29	28	27	25	24
238	69	64	59	55	51	48	45	42	40	37	35	33	32	30	28	27	26	24
242	70	65	60	56	52	49	46	43	40	38	36	34	32	30	29	28	26	25
246	72	66	61	57	53	50	47	44	41	39	37	35	33	31	29	28	27	25
251	73	67	63	58	54	51	47	45	42	39	37	35	33	32	30	29	27	26
255	74	69	64	59	55	52	48	45	43	40	38	36	34	32	31	29	28	26
260	76	70	65	60	56	52	49	46	43	41	39	36	34	33	31	30	28	27
264	77	71	66	61	57	53	50	47	44	42	39	37	35	33	32	30	29	27
268	78	72	67	62	58	54	51	48	45	42	40	38	36	34	32	31	29	28
273	79	73	68	63	59	55	52	48	46	43	40	38	36	34	33	31	30	28
277	81	75	69	64	60	56	52	49	46	44	41	39	37	35	33	32	30	29
282	82	76	70	65	61	57	53	50	47	44	42	40	37	35	34	32	30	29
286	83	77	71	66	62	58	54	51	48	45	42	40	38	36	34	33	31	29
290	84	78	72	67	63	59	55	52	48	46	43	41	39	37	35	33	31	30
295	86	79	74	68	64	60	56	52	49	46	44	41	39	37	35	34	32	30
299	87	80	75	69	65	60	57	53	50	47	44	42	40	38	36	34	32	31
304	88	82	76	70	66	61	57	54	51	48	45	43	40	38	36	35	33	31
308	90	83	77	71	67	62	58	55	51	48	46	43	41	39	37	35	33	32
312	91	84	78	72	68	63	59	55	52	49	46	44	41	39	37	36	34	32

Body Mass Index

Underweight (<19)

Desirable (19–25)

Increased health risks (25–30)

Obese (30–40)

Extremely obese (>40)

Source: Expert Panel on the Identification, Evaluation, and Treatment of Overweight in Adults, 1998.

It's In Your Genes

Genes influence potential, but they don't assure it. The 30,000 genes that form the blueprint of the human body are subject to the influence of the environment and behavior. It's true that part of your makeup is a given and cannot be changed; even that part, however, interacts with the environment. Because of our different genetic blueprints, each person experiences different results when engaging in aerobic training. For instance, one person might see a faster improvement in performance than another person does after the same amount of training. Such differences often derive from different genetic makeups.

To reach your genetic potential in fitness, you first have to "switch on" your genes by training. Genes carry the code for the production of proteins. When you do aerobic activity, you activate or "turn on" specific genes located in your muscle fibers (another term for muscle cells). This activation causes a messenger molecule to exit the nucleus of the muscle cell, bind to another chemical that creates protein, and tell that chemical which protein, or enzyme, to make. These enzymes, in turn, help your muscles use fat and carbohydrate. Without aerobic activity, none of this happens, so you can see that being active is very important. Even if you are genetically gifted, you cannot reach your potential if you don't train!

Responses Vary

Aerobic endurance training generally leads to a 20 to 25 percent increase in aerobic fitness (even more when accompanied by weight loss), but the response is variable. Dr. Claude Bouchard found that improvements in aerobic fitness ranged from 0 to 41 percent for 10 pairs of identical twins. In his study, 77 percent of the variation in the response to training was dependent on genes. Clearly, then, hered- ity plays a major role in our ability to respond to training. Other factors that may influ- ence your response to training include maturation, nutrition (energy and amino acids needed to build protein), adequate rest, and even chemical-related emotional factors such as stress or depression. Your response to training is also affected by the intensity and duration of your training (more on this in the next chapter).

Training (intensity, duration, frequency), maturation, nutrition, rest, and stress 23%

Genes 77%

Factors that influence your response to training.

Keys to Aerobic Fitness

➤ To improve your aerobic fitness, do activities in which you use large muscles (as in walking, running, cycling, swimming).

➤ Training is specific—decide what you are training for, then train in that specific activity.

➤ Aerobic endurance training improves your heart and lung function, burns lots of fat, and improves delivery of oxygen to your muscles.

➤ Genes influence potential, but they don't assure it. Do what you can to approach your potential.

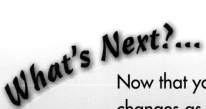

What's Next?...

Now that you know how your body changes as it becomes aerobically fit, move on to chapter 3 to learn *how* to train for aerobic fitness.

3

Aerobic
Fitness
Training

A Gentle Pastime

We should approach training not as if we are trying to smash our way through some enormous wall, but as "a gentle pastime by which we coax a slow, continuous stream of adaptations out of the body."

~ Ned Frederick (quoted portion)

Jacob

is in his late 20s.

He put on weight during his first year in college (the "freshman 15," in American parlance) and kept adding a little weight each year. He liked his life of watching television and enjoying occasional nights of dancing at bars, but he wasn't feeling great about how he looked, and he felt sluggish all day long. To address the issue, he started a simple fitness program several months ago. He hadn't been active for a long time, so at first he simply took his dog on a walk every other night.

...he noticed he was sleeping better

The first night, he went only a few blocks, but he felt better afterward, so he started adding distance to his walking sessions. Soon he was walking for half an hour every night on a route that combined city streets and a walking trail near his apartment complex. In time, he noticed that he was sleeping better and getting some attention from potential romantic partners. Now, Jacob incorporates some jogging into his walk on a couple of nights each week. On Saturdays, he goes for a longer walk, plays fetch with his dog in a field by the walking trail, and even meets up with some buddies from work to play pickup basketball—something he never would have done only a few months ago. He's trimmed down, and he's happy with the way he looks and feels. During a recent walk, he met an active young woman. They are now dating regularly and are planning a summer hiking trip in the mountains.

Going Farther

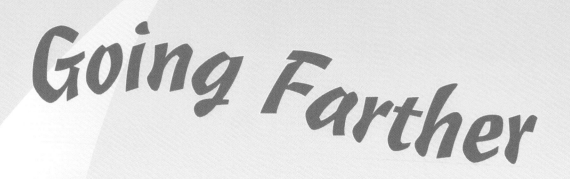

Training activates genes to form new protein. Aerobic endurance training leads to an increase in the oxidative powerhouses called mitochondria and in the protein enzymes that derive energy from carbohydrate and fat. You stimulate these changes when you overload the muscles used in a given activity. Overload is accomplished by going a bit farther, or a bit faster, or both farther and faster than you usually do. This, in a nutshell, is the essence of training.

LESS
FIT

Aerobic training leads to an increased density of mitochondria in muscle tissue.

Gently train by going a bit farther and a bit faster, and feel your level of energy increase.

MORE
FIT

and Faster

How to Adjust Your Aerobic Fitness Training

This chapter shows you how to coax important adaptations from your body. I will tell you how to train while enjoying the process. You can create a prescription for exercise by controlling the intensity, duration, and frequency of your training. Whether you are a newcomer, an active person looking to improve your fitness, or someone who is already very fit, this chapter provides a prescription for you.

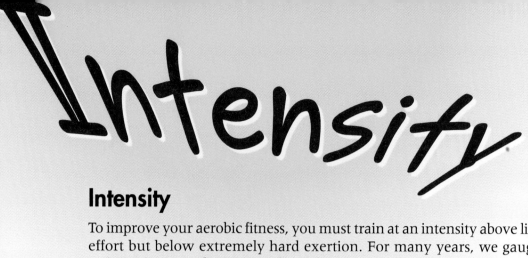

Intensity

To improve your aerobic fitness, you must train at an intensity above light effort but below extremely hard exertion. For many years, we gauged training intensity by means of exercise heart rate, and this approach led people to believe that the goal of training was to raise the heart rate, but that isn't the case. The true purpose of training is to engage a large muscle mass in sustained activity that is fueled by the oxidation of fat and carbohydrate. With this in mind—and in view of the fact that heart rate varies considerably between individuals—we will use the rating of perceived exertion (RPE) as an indicator of training intensity.

Evaluating Your Intensity Based on Heart Rate, Breathing, and Duration

Estimated heart rate	Breathing scale	Duration
60		
70	Can sing full songs	Could continue all day
80		Could continue 4–8 hours
90	Can sing partial verses	Could continue 3–4 hours
100		Could continue 2–3 hours
110	Can talk in full sentences	Could continue 1–2 hours
120		Could continue 45–60 minutes
130	Can talk in short sentences	Could continue 30–45 minutes
140		Could continue 20–30 minutes
150	Breathing hard, thinking clearly	Could continue 15–20 minutes
160		Could continue 10–15 minutes
170	Breathing very hard	Could continue 5–10 minutes
180		Could continue 2–5 minutes
190		Could continue 1–2 minutes
200		Could continue <1 minute

Adapted by permission from Sharkey and Gaskill, 2007, p. 103.

Developed by Swedish psychologist Gunnar Borg, the RPE scale allows you to determine the appropriate intensity of effort. The scale ranges from 6 to 20, with 6 indicating no exertion at all and 20 indicating maximal exertion. Ratings of 7 to 12 are considered light, 13 and 14 are somewhat hard, and 15 to 19 are progressively harder. The table on page 46 shows how the ratings might correspond to heart rate, breathing, and duration. The breathing scale helps you gauge the effort, and the duration scale lets you know how long you could continue at that pace. The numbers on the perceived exertion scale are also related to exercise heart rate; add a zero to the rating number (which I've done in the first column of the table) to approximate your heart rate during exercise. Longer training sessions can be done at 11 to 13 on the scale, whereas shorter workouts may be done in the 14 to 16 range. If you are an athlete training for a race, brief periods (intervals) of exertion may be done at 17 and 18 on the RPE scale, or 5 to 10 minutes (for a rating of 17) or 2 to 5 minutes (for a rating of 18) on the duration scale.

Intensity is important if you are training to improve your performance in a sport (e.g., running). But if your goal is to increase your endurance or stamina, improve your health, or maintain a healthy body weight, then your training should emphasize duration.

DURATION

Duration

Duration and intensity of exercise go together; if you increase one, you necessarily decrease the other. Duration can be considered in terms of time, distance, or calories used, and these three factors are of course related. I like to focus, however, on calories, because doing so is educational. You can easily see how many calories you consume when you eat and drink simply by looking at food and beverage labels; a light beer, for instance, provides about 100 calories. You can then use this information to determine how much of a given kind of exercise it will take to balance your energy intake. For example, since jogging 1 mile (1.6 km) typically uses more than 100 calories, you would need to jog just under a mile to burn the calories consumed in that light beer. This approach makes you think about what you eat and drink—and what you will have to do to achieve balance between your energy intake and your energy expenditure.

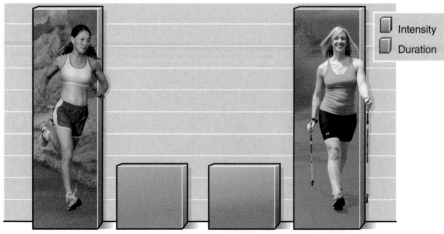

Intensity
Duration

To boost performance in sport, increase intensity.

To boost stamina and maintain body weight, increase duration.

What Is a Calorie?

The calorie (technically, a kilocalorie) is a unit of energy; more specifically, a calorie is defined as the amount of heat required to raise the temperature of 1 kilogram of water (1 liter) by 1 degree Celsius. When we eat, we store calories; when we exercise, we burn them, and the number of calories you burn during exercise is influenced by how much you weigh. A heavier person burns more calories while running at a certain pace than does a lighter person. In this book, caloric expenditures are based on a weight of 150 pounds (68 kg); you can adjust the figures to fit yourself by adding or subtracting 10 percent for every 15 pounds (6.8 kg) over or under 150 pounds. For example, when running, a 150-pound person will expend approximately 113 calories per mile (1.6 km). If you weigh 165 pounds (75 kg), add 10 percent to the 113 calories in order to determine how many calories you would burn while running a mile (113 × 0.10 = 11.3 + 113 = 124.3 calories).

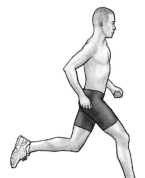

135 pounds (61 kg)
113 x .10 = 11.3
113 - 11.3 = 101.7 calories
       burned per mile
       (1.6 km)

150 pounds (68 kg)
113 calories burned
per mile (1.6 km)

165 pounds (75 kg)
113 x .10 = 11.3
113 + 11.3 =124.3 calories
       burned per mile
       (1.6 km)

See the appendix on page 304 for a listing of activities and the number of calories (depending on your body weight) you can burn by doing them.

FitFact

Duration can be measured in time, distance, or calories burned: Your walk might last 30 minutes, cover 2 miles (3.2 km), or burn 200 calories.

The table below offers information to help you choose the duration of your aerobic fitness training.

Duration of Training

Fitness level	Walk/jog distance	Calories burned*
Beginner	1–2 miles (1.6–3.2 km)	100–200
Intermediate	2–4 miles (3.2–6.4 km)	200–400
Advanced	>4 miles (>6.4 km)	>400

*For every 15 pounds above or below 150 pounds (or every 7 kg above or below 68 kg), add or subtract 10 percent.

Adapted by permission from Sharkey and Gaskill, 2007, p. 106.

Can Sing Partial Verses ▶ Use the **beginner** fitness level if you are just starting out or have been physically active for less than 6 weeks. Using the breathing scale in the table on page 46, you should be able to sing partial verses as you walk 1 to 2 miles (1.6 to 3.2 km).

Can Talk in Full Sentences ▶ Follow the guidelines for the **intermediate** fitness level if you are regularly active for 30 minutes a day on 5 or more days of the week and can walk 2 miles (3.2 km) at a brisk pace without batting an eye. You should be able to talk in full sentences as you walk or jog 2 to 4 miles (3.2 to 6.4 km).

Can Talk in Short Sentences ▶ Select the prescription for the **advanced** fitness level if you have been active for more than 6 months and can walk 4 miles (6.4 km) without difficulty. You should be able to talk in short sentences as you walk 4 or more miles.

If your preferred activity is something other than walking or jogging, see the appendix. You can find more training guidelines in chapter 4.

Frequency

Low-fit individuals can improve their aerobic fitness by doing three training sessions a week on alternating days. However, if they want to continue improving their fitness as their training progresses in intensity and duration, they must also increase their frequency of training. Changes in fitness are, in fact, directly related to frequency of training, and training on 6 days per week is much more effective than training on 3 days. Thus, if your goal is fitness or weight control, consider exercising more frequently. Athletes, of course, train hard. They perform long training sessions, or train two or more times a day, on 2 or 3 days a week. But they also observe the hard–easy principle, meaning that they

FitFact

More frequent exercise will increase fitness and weight control—but don't overtrain!

51

follow hard or long sessions with easy or short ones. The human body needs time to respond to the stimulus of training—to make the proteins stimulated by training. If you don't allow your body adequate time to recover from training, you won't get the most out of your training program. In fact, overtraining can lead to poor performance, overuse injury, and even illness (it can suppress your immune system).

Experiment with schedules to find one that suits you. Work out daily if you prefer, or try an every-other-day plan and increase the duration. Whatever you do, be sure to schedule at least one day of relative rest or diversion each week. Remember Ned Frederick's view of training as a "gentle pastime through which we coax a . . . stream of adaptations out of the body." Use the following table to guide you in deciding how often to be active.

Frequency of Training

Fitness level	Frequency (days/week)
Beginner	3 or 4
Intermediate	5 or 6
Advanced	6+*

*Athletes sometimes do two sessions per day, but they always follow a hard day with an easy day.
Adapted by permission from Sharkey and Gaskill, 2007, p. 107.

Now that we've discussed intensity, duration, and frequency, it's time to put all the factors together in your personalized prescription for fitness. See the table below to help guide your decisions.

Aerobic Fitness Prescription

Fitness level	RPE	Duration (calories)*	Frequency (days/week)	Walk/jog distance (miles)
Beginner	11–13	100–200	3 or 4	1–2 (1.6–3.2 km)
Intermediate	12–14	200–400	4 or 5	2–4 (3.2–6.4 km)
Advanced	13–15	>400	6	>4 (>6.4 km)

*Estimate 100 calories per mile (1.6 km) of brisk walking or jogging.
Adapted by permission from Sharkey and Gaskill, 2007, p. 107.

This is a basic guide to fitness training—a place to start. Since the benefits plateau when you remain at the same level of exercise, you must progress in duration, in frequency, and, eventually, in intensity if you want to continue making progress.

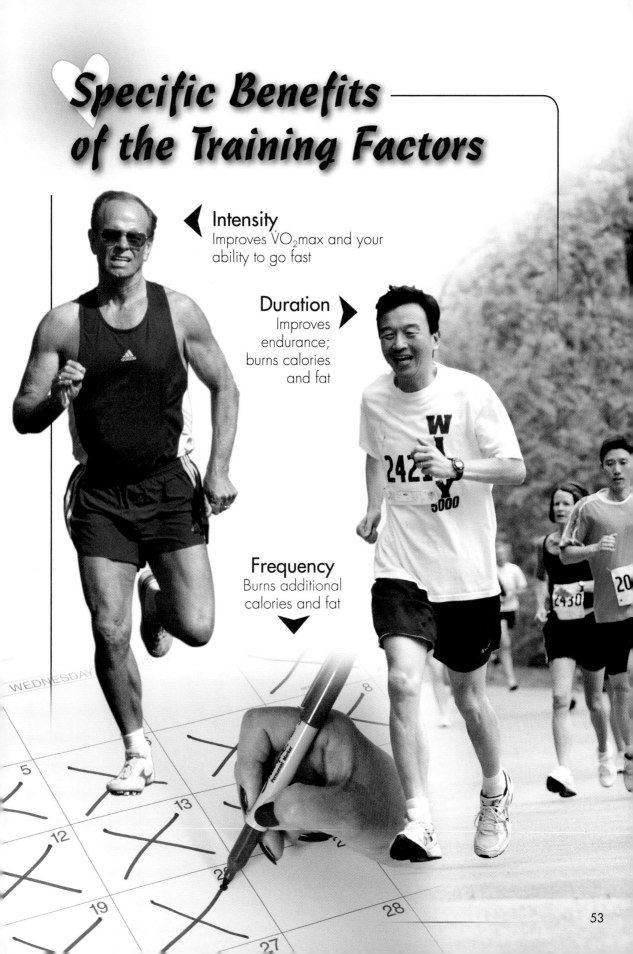

Specific Benefits of the Training Factors

Intensity
Improves $\dot{V}O_2$max and your ability to go fast

Duration
Improves endurance; burns calories and fat

Frequency
Burns additional calories and fat

Progression

As you coax that "gentle stream" of improvements from your body, it pays to remember the adage "Make haste slowly." In other words, proceed deliberately for best results. In training, *progression* refers to how we gradually increase the overall training load. Gradual progress gives your body time to rest, recover, and adjust to the demands of training. You can meet your health goal by doing 30 to 60 minutes of moderate activity on most days of the week; thus, a brisk walk can help you meet this goal. If you have been sedentary, however, you may have to become active before you begin to train.

Follow these guidelines to gradually increase your training load:

Increase a session 100 to 200 calories, or 1 to 2 miles (1.6–3.2 km) above what you have been doing, while staying at a comfortable pace. Each week, include a short training session, an intermediate session, and a longer one.

Be willing to adjust your daily training plan. If you are tired, reduce the load by going shorter, easier, or maybe not at all.

6. Pay attention to your body

1. Increase duration

2. Increase frequency

Add a day with a short or intermediate workout at a comfortable pace.

5. Repeat the cycle

3. Increase intensity

4. Rest when necessary

Build on your progress and slowly increase duration, frequency, and intensity until you feel you are where you would like to be.

After increasing duration, frequency, and intensity over several weeks, schedule an easier week for recovery.

Replace an intermediate-length workout with one that is slightly more intense (RPE 13–15). Try increasing your pace for 5 to 10 minutes, and then slowing down to recover; repeat several times. Add increased-intensity sessions gradually, paying attention to how your body responds. When you increase intensity (i.e., move to a higher level of perceived exertion), reduce the duration of the workout.

♥ Neck Check

Should you train when you have a respiratory tract infection? To answer this question, Dr. Randy Eichner recommends the neck check.

Symptoms *above* the neck:

Stuffy nose
Sneezing
Scratchy throat

Give your workout a try at half speed. If you feel better after 10 minutes, you can increase your pace and finish the workout.

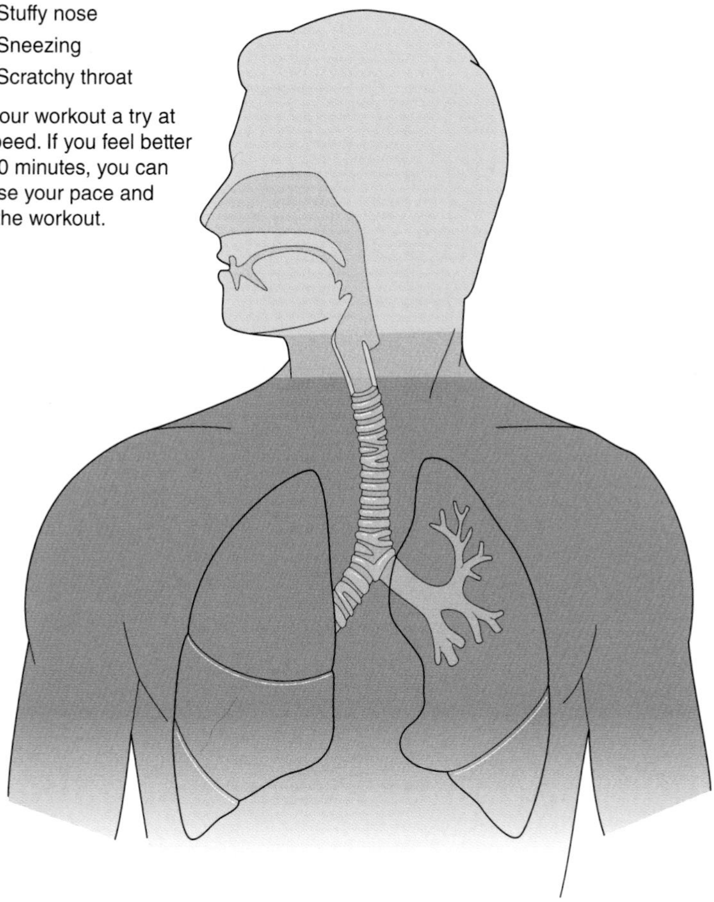

Symptoms *below* the neck:

Aching muscles
Coughing
Fever
Nausea
Diarrhea

Take the day off. You can return to training when your fever has been gone for at least 24 hours without the aid of fever-reducing medication.

Great Expectations

After a few weeks of training, you will notice that the "slow, continuous stream of adaptations" you've coaxed from your body allows you to go faster or farther than you did before training. After several months of training, the awkward mile of jogging has evolved into an easy 4-mile (6.4 km) run. Once again, the key to these achievements is to *make haste slowly*. If, instead, you rush the process, you may end up experiencing pain, injury, or illness. Take your time. Your performance *will* improve within a month. You'll experience improved energy and vigor, and you'll begin to feel better about yourself and your body.

On average, aerobic fitness ($\dot{V}O_2$max) improves by 25 percent after several months—even more for those who lose weight—and improvements are generally greater for those who start from a lower level of fitness. One's ability to perform submaximal work (less than the maximum of which a person is capable) such as hiking, jogging, cycling, and swimming continues to improve for many months. As a result, a once-sedentary individual can develop the capacity to climb a mountain or run a marathon. As you progress, you can sustain an increasing percentage of your maximal capacity and thus continue once-wearying activities indefinitely without experiencing undue fatigue. These capacities are represented by the middle and bottom lines in the graph below. Notice that they continue to gradually climb. What's more, these benefits reach beyond your training sessions into all of your daily activities. Along the way, you gain access to body fat as a source of energy, thus making it easier to maintain a trim, pleasing figure. Thus, fitness, this gentle pastime, expands your horizons and improves your health.

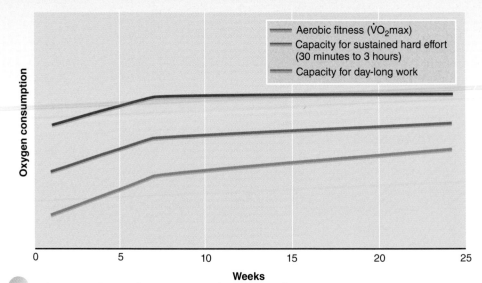

Initial training brings big gains. With prolonged training, your maximum aerobic fitness will begin to level off, but your capacity to perform at lower levels will continue to improve.

Choosing an Activity

Remember from chapter 2 that in order to train well, you must first decide what you are training for. Overall fitness, good health, and enhanced appearance may be worthy goals, but they do not provide a framework for training. This is the case because training is specific; it addresses the muscles used in a given activity. Thus, you must select an activity that will help you meet your goals. Above all, that activity must be meaningful and enjoyable to you!

Aerobic training involves rhythmic, large-muscle activities such as walking, running (jogging), cycling, swimming, cross-country skiing, and rowing. Such activities demand that your body sustain increases in respiration, circulation, and muscle metabolism; as a result, they lead to adaptations in the muscles and systems involved. Select one or more activities that you enjoy and will continue to engage in— perhaps for a lifetime.

Walking may be the most versatile aerobic exercise. It can be done almost anywhere, costs little, and can even save you money. Walking is a worthy end in itself, but it is even more compelling if you do it with a significant other, a friend, or a dog. Dr. William Morgan, an eminent sport psychologist, has studied lifelong adherents to activity and found two meaningful catego-ries for which walking fills the bill: transportation and walking the dog. Aerobic training prepares you for extended hikes in national parks or wilderness areas or for foreign travel, and it builds the foundation for independent living as a senior citizen. To improve your performance, start at a comfortable pace, and then gradually add distance, frequency, and, finally, intensity.

Running or jogging was my preferred exercise for many years. It is versatile and inexpensive and provides a great way to explore locations that you visit for business or travel. It can also be sustained for decades—if you do it in moderation. My advice is to cross-train with other activities (e.g., cycling) in order to minimize the wear and tear on your joints. If the idea appeals to you, running also prepares you to participate in fun runs and road races.

Cycling offers a less traumatic way to train. Bicycling builds your leg strength and your endurance and thus provides a great way to cross-train for hikers and runners. Mountain bikes allow you to get off the beaten path, whereas road and touring bikes take you down country roads, and commuting bikes let you ride to work. And, as with running, if you're interested, cycling can prepare you to do longer activities—in this case, extended bicycle trips or endurance rides, such as century rides of 100 miles (160 km).

FitFact

Above all, choose an activity that is meaningful and enjoyable to you.

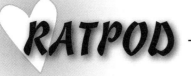

RATPOD

The RATPOD is a 1-day charity ride to support Camp Mak-A-Dream (a camp for children and adults with cancer) that covers 156 miles (251 km) while crossing two mountain passes and several sizable hills. The title stands for Ride Around The Pioneers in One Day (the Pioneer Mountains are located in southwestern Montana). At my advanced age, it takes me 12 hours to complete the ride. Why volunteer to do such a demanding ride? Beyond the fact that it's for a good cause, it motivates me to engage in several months of training that provides significant health benefits. I train with a friend and do group rides with our local cycling club.

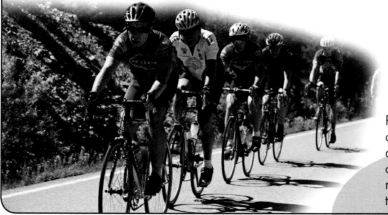

Participating in an organized event, as these RATPOD cyclists did, can motivate you to train.

Swimming is a wonderful aerobic activity for those who possess the skill and have access to a training site. It is easy on the body and can be done well into the eighth decade of life. Swim training prepares you to swim faster and farther. Is it the ideal activity because it involves most of the muscles in the body? Not necessarily. The ideal activity is the one you look forward to doing on a regular basis—possibly for the rest of your life.

Cross-country skiing is one of my favorite ways to keep active. Like swimming, it utilizes the arms and legs and thus allows you to burn more calories with no greater sense of effort. It also provides the opportunity to enjoy beautiful winter days when others are forced to exercise indoors. Use cross-country skiing to prepare for ski tours, citizen races, or even a ski marathon (50 km, or 31 mi).

Paddling in a canoe or kayak is another wonderful outdoor activity. With appropriate training, you will be able to paddle comfortably for hours. Eventually, you will be fit enough for an extended trip in the Boundary Waters Canoe Area (in Minnesota) or a backcountry area near you.

Skating is another activity that can be performed outdoors. In-line skates can be used as a mode of transportation, and during the winter you can enjoy using ice skates or skating skis.

Outdoor Activity

You might elect to walk or jog on a treadmill or ride a stationary bicycle indoors. When possible, however, do your activity outdoors. There's nothing better than doing the same activity outdoors on a sunny day. Walk or run in the park or on a river trail; the changing scenery even helps pass the time more quickly. Learn to cope with the weather. If you learn to manage the quality of your exercise experience, you are more likely to persist.

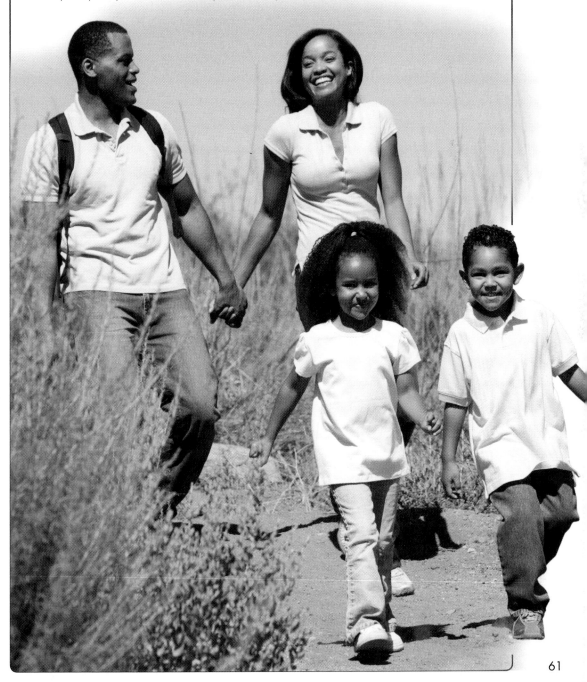

Choosing an Activity

In chapter 4, you will find sample training programs for walking, jogging and running, cycling, and swimming. Before considering them, however, you need to choose the activity that will suit you best. Use this checklist to help you select the activity that you will try first.

❑ **Walking**

➤ This is a good first step if you have not been active in a long time.

➤ Walking is a great option if you don't have access to a pool or don't like to swim, and if you are not comfortable on a bicycle.

➤ Walking requires very little equipment—just a good pair of shoes will do it.

➤ You may like the freedom that walking provides: You can do it anytime, anyplace.

❑ **Jogging**

➤ You're already somewhat fit and want to do something more intense than walking. Check out the walk–jog or jog–run programs presented in chapter 4.

➤ You can't cycle or swim due to equipment, setting, or skill reasons.

❑ **Running**

➤ Your knees are healthy, and you'd like the higher intensity of this activity.

➤ You can walk briskly at a pace of 15 minutes per mile (9.3 min per km) and you like the idea of stepping it up.

➤ You have friends who run and sometimes participate in fun runs.

➤ The idea of joining a running club appeals to you. Check the Web or go to your local (running) shoe store for information.

❑ **Cycling**

➤ Walking is too tame for you, but knee problems keep you from running.

➤ You have the means to borrow or purchase a good bike.

➤ You like meeting new people. Check the Web or go to your local bicycle store to learn about cycling clubs and cycling events in your community.

➤ You love the idea of moving quickly through the countryside with a tailwind sustaining your pace or a headwind offering a challenge.

❑ **Swimming**

➤ You have access to a pool and will be able to get to the pool regularly.

➤ You really enjoy the activity of swimming.

➤ You love the coolness of the water and the challenge of moving your body against its resistance.

➤ You have the skill or can take a class to develop your swimming technique.

Keys to Aerobic Fitness Training

➤ Increase duration first.

➤ Increase frequency second.

➤ Increase intensity gradually.

➤ When you add intensity, reduce duration.

➤ Use the hard–easy principle: Follow hard or long sessions with easy or short ones.

➤ Pay attention to your body. Rest when you need to.

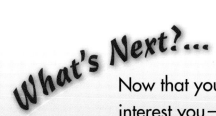

Now that you know what aerobic activities interest you—and how far and fast you might go—you're ready to design your own aerobic fitness training program. Move on to chapter 4 to learn how.

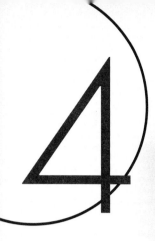

4

Aerobic Programs

Have It Your Way

Opportunity is
missed by most
people because
it is dressed in
overalls and looks
like work.

~ Thomas Alva Edison

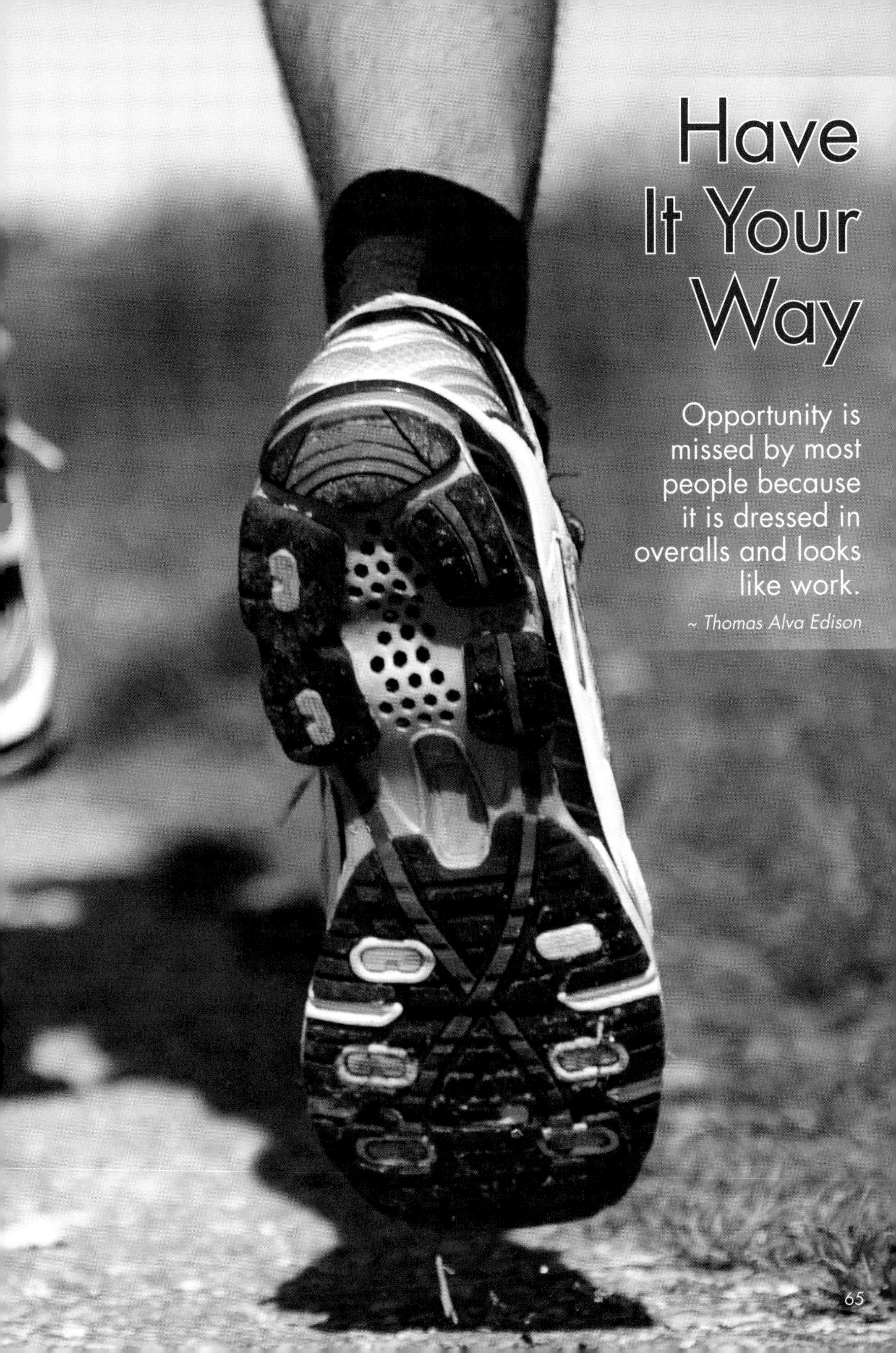

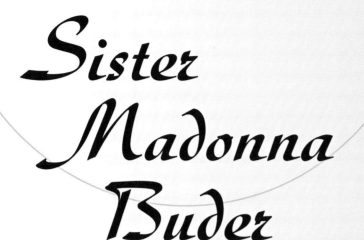

Sister Madonna Buder

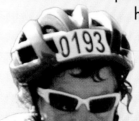

was 48 years old when a priest recommended the potential of physical activity, especially running, which has the power to temper depression and harmonize the mind, body, and soul. She started running but didn't enter a race until she heard of a family member having personal problems,

Sister Madonna Buder

...harmonize the mind, body, and soul

after which she dedicated her effort in the Spokane, Washington, 8.2-mile (13.2 km) Bloomsday Run to that cause. Next, she set her sights on the Boston Marathon, running with the bishop's approval, to raise money for the fight against multiple sclerosis. Then she saw a story about triathlons, and, having enjoyed biking and swimming, she decided to give it a try. After she finished a local short triathlon, she moved on to longer events and eventually set out to qualify for the Ironman Triathlon, which entails doing a 2.4-mile (3.9 km) swim, a 112-mile (180.2 km) bike ride, and a full marathon run (26.2 miles [42.2 km]). She qualified and was off to Hawaii for her first Ironman race. She has since completed the Ironman distance more than 35 times, setting a record in the female 75 to 79 age group!

Personalize Your

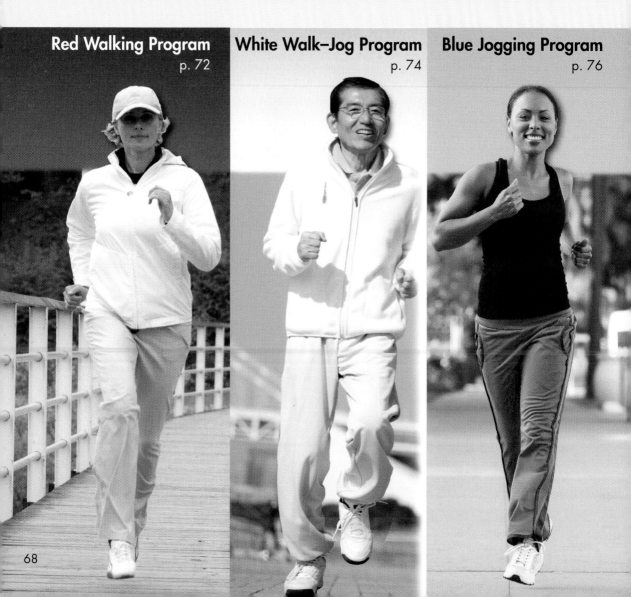

The simplest training program is the one you design to fit the rhythm of your life—one that is meaningful to you. You can walk a little farther on one day and a little faster on another, and you can take it easy on the third day. As your fitness improves, you can add a longer walk on the weekend. It really is that simple. But since many folks prefer more

Red Walking Program
p. 72

White Walk–Jog Program
p. 74

Blue Jogging Program
p. 76

Training Program

direction, I provide walk–jog–run programs, along with bicycling and swimming programs. The walk–jog programs are ideal for those making the transition to fitness. The jog–run, cycling, and swimming programs illustrate the elements of training for those in higher fitness categories.

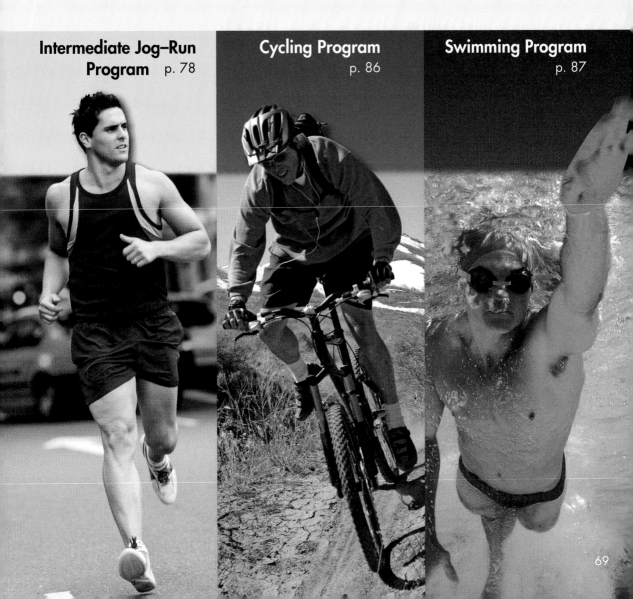

Intermediate Jog–Run Program p. 78

Cycling Program p. 86

Swimming Program p. 87

Starter Program (Walk–Jog)

The starter program, which includes the red, white, and blue walking and jogging programs, was prepared by the President's Council on Physical Fitness and Sports. Take the walk test to determine your exercise level.

Walk Test

Use the walk test to determine how many minutes (up to 10) you can walk at a brisk pace on a level surface without undue difficulty or discomfort. Try it: Put on some walking shoes and find a safe, level surface to walk on. This might be a sidewalk in your neighborhood or near your workplace or a track at a local school or community center. Start walking at a brisk pace and stop after 10 minutes—or before that if you reach a point where you cannot continue.

➤ If you cannot walk for 5 minutes, begin with the red walking program.

➤ If you can walk for more than 5 minutes but fewer than 10, begin with the third week of the red walking program.

➤ If you can walk for 10 minutes but are somewhat tired afterward, start with the white walk–jog program.

➤ If you can walk for the full 10 minutes comfortably, then you're ready for a more demanding workout. The next step is to take the 10-minute walk–jog test (but wait until the next day so you're fresh).

Walk–Jog Test

This test calls for you to alternately walk 50 steps (i.e., each foot strikes the ground 25 times), and then jog 50 steps. Continue this alternating process for 10 minutes. Pace your walking portions at 120 steps per minute (i.e., your left foot strikes the ground at 1-second intervals). Pace your jogging portions at 144 steps per minute (your left foot strikes the ground 18 times every 15 seconds).

➤ If you cannot complete the 10-minute walk–jog test, start with the third week of the white walk–jog program.

➤ If you can complete the 10-minute walk–jog test but are tired and winded afterward, begin with the last week of the white walk–jog program, and then move on to the blue jogging program.

➤ If you can perform the 10-minute walk–jog test comfortably, then you're ready to start with the blue jogging program.

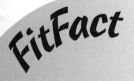

FitFact

Before starting an aerobic fitness training program, test your level of fitness so that you know where to start.

RED WALKING PROGRAM

In this program, you walk every other day (see the table on the following page). During week 1, you walk briskly (rating of perceived exertion, or RPE, is equal to 10 or 11 on the scale of 6 to 20) for 5 minutes, or for a shorter time if you become uncomfortably tired. Next, shift gears and walk slowly for 3 minutes, and then walk briskly again for 5 minutes or until you become uncomfortably tired. During week 2 of the program, you use the same sequence but increase your pace as soon as you can walk 5 minutes without soreness or fatigue. During week 3, increase the duration of your brisk walking to 8 minutes; then, during week 4, increase your pace. At that point, you will be ready to move on to week 1 of the white walk–jog program.

Red Walking Program

Week	Sunday	Monday	Tuesday	Wednesday	Thursday	Friday	Saturday
1	Brisk walk 5 min	Off	Brisk walk 5 min	Off	Brisk walk 5 min	Off	Brisk walk 5 min
	Slow walk (or rest) 3 min		Slow walk (or rest) 3 min		Slow walk (or rest) 3 min		Slow walk (or rest) 3 min
	Brisk walk 5 min		Brisk walk 5 min		Brisk walk 5 min		Brisk walk 5 min
2	Off	Brisk walk 5 min	Off	Brisk walk 5 min	Off	Brisk walk 5 min	Off
		Slow walk (or rest) 3 min		Slow walk (or rest) 3 min		Slow walk (or rest) 3 min	
		Brisk walk 5 min		Brisk walk 5 min		Brisk walk 5 min	
3	Brisk walk 8 min	Off	Brisk walk 8 min	Off	Brisk walk 8 min	Off	Brisk walk 8 min
	Slow walk (or rest) 3 min		Slow walk (or rest) 3 min		Slow walk (or rest) 3 min		Slow walk (or rest) 3 min
	Brisk walk 8 min		Brisk walk 8 min		Brisk walk 8 min		Brisk walk 8 min
4	Off	Brisk walk 8 min	Off	Brisk walk 8 min	Off	Brisk walk 8 min	Off
		Slow walk (or rest) 3 min		Slow walk (or rest) 3 min		Slow walk (or rest) 3 min	
		Brisk walk 8 min		Brisk walk 8 min		Brisk walk 8 min	

Reprinted by permission from Sharkey and Gaskill, 2007, p. 119, as adapted from President's Council on Physical Fitness and Sports, 1975.

WHITE WALK–JOG PROGRAM

YOU begin this program by walking briskly for 10 minutes, or for a shorter time if you become uncomfortably tired (see the table on the following page). Then, after a brief stint of slow walking to allow your body to recover, you'll resume the brisk pace. During week 2, you will increase the duration of your brisk walking, and week 3 will bring you up to about 30 minutes of walking on most days of the week, which is the minimum level of activity suggested by the American College of Sports Medicine in order to achieve health benefits. During week 4, you'll incorporate short jogs. You'll jog for 10 seconds, walk for a minute to recover, and repeat 11 times. You'll then increase your jogging during week 5. You'll be active on at least 4 days of each week. Once you've done the 5 weeks of the white walk–jog program, you're ready to begin week 1 of the blue jogging program.

White Walk–Jog Program

Week	Sunday	Monday	Tuesday	Wednesday	Thursday	Friday	Saturday
1	Brisk walk 10 min Slow walk (or rest) 3 min Brisk walk 10 min	Brisk walk 10 min Slow walk (or rest) 3 min Brisk walk 10 min	Off	Brisk walk 10 min Slow walk (or rest) 3 min Brisk walk 10 min	Off	Brisk walk 10 min Slow walk (or rest) 3 min Brisk walk 10 min	Off
2	Brisk walk 15 min Slow walk (or rest) 3 min Brisk walk 10 min	Off	Brisk walk 15 min Slow walk (or rest) 3 min Brisk walk 10 min	Off	Brisk walk 15 min Slow walk (or rest) 3 min Brisk walk 15 min	Off	Brisk walk 15 min Slow walk (or rest) 3 min Brisk walk 15 min
3	Brisk walk 10 min Rest 3 min Brisk walk 15 min	Moderate walk 30 min	Brisk walk 10 min Rest 3 min Brisk walk 15 min	Moderate walk 30 min	Brisk walk 10 min Rest 3 min Brisk walk 15 min	Moderate walk 30 min	Off
4	Jog 10 sec (25 yd) Walk 1 min (100 yd) 12×	Off	Jog 10 sec (25 yd) Walk 1 min (100 yd) 12×	Off	Jog 10 sec (25 yd) Walk 1 min (100 yd) 12×	Off	Jog 10 sec (25 yd) Walk 1 min (100 yd) 12×
5	Off	Jog 20 sec (50 yd) Walk 1 min (100 yd) 12×	Off	Jog 20 sec (50 yd) Walk 1 min (100 yd) 12×	Off	Jog 20 sec (50 yd) Walk 1 min (100 yd) 12×	Jog 20 sec (50 yd) Walk 1 min (100 yd) 12×

Walk briskly at an RPE of 10 or 11. Jog at an RPE of 13 to 15. Meters = yards $\times$ 0.91.

Reprinted by permission from Sharkey and Gaskill, 2007, p. 120, as adapted from President's Council on Physical Fitness and Sports, 1975.

BLUE JOGGING PROGRAM

In this program, you are active 5 days per week and you increase the duration of your jogging each week (see the table on the following page). Consider the fact that although 30 minutes is the minimum amount of time needed to achieve health benefits through exercise, the Institute of Medicine has recommended 1 full hour of daily activity in order to achieve *greater* health benefits and maintain healthy body weight. With this in mind, once you have completed the 8-week blue jogging program, you may want to consider moving on to the intermediate jog–run program.

Blue Jogging Program

Week	Sunday	Monday	Tuesday	Wednesday	Thursday	Friday	Saturday
1	Jog 40 sec (100 yd) Walk 1 min (100 yd) 9×	Jog 40 sec (100 yd) Walk 1 min (100 yd) 9×	Off	Jog 40 sec (100 yd) Walk 1 min (100 yd) 9×	Jog 40 sec (100 yd) Walk 1 min (100 yd) 9×	Off	Jog 40 sec (100 yd) Walk 1 min (100 yd) 9×
2	Jog 1 min (150 yd) Walk 1 min (100 yd) 8×	Jog 1 min (150 yd) Walk 1 min (100 yd) 8×	Jog 1 min (150 yd) Walk 1 min (100 yd) 8×	Off	Jog 1 min (150 yd) Walk 1 min (100 yd) 8×	Jog 1 min (150 yd) Walk 1 min (100 yd) 8×	Off
3	Jog 2 min (300 yd) Walk 1 min (100 yd) 6×	Jog 2 min (300 yd) Walk 1 min (100 yd) 6×	Off	Jog 2 min (300 yd) Walk 1 min (100 yd) 6×	Jog 2 min (300 yd) Walk 1 min (100 yd) 6×	Off	Jog 2 min (300 yd) Walk 1 min (100 yd) 6×
4	Jog 4 min (600 yd) Walk 1 min (100 yd) 4×	Off	Jog 4 min (600 yd) Walk 1 min (100 yd) 4×	Jog 4 min (600 yd) Walk 1 min (100 yd) 4×	Off	Jog 4 min (600 yd) Walk 1 min (100 yd) 4×	Jog 4 min (600 yd) Walk 1 min (100 yd) 4×
5	Jog 6 min (900 yd) Walk 1 min (100 yd) 3×	Jog 6 min (900 yd) Walk 1 min (100 yd) 3×	Off	Jog 6 min (900 yd) Walk 1 min (100 yd) 3×	Jog 6 min (900 yd) Walk 1 min (100 yd) 3×	Off	Jog 6 min (900 yd) Walk 1 min (100 yd) 3×
6	Jog 8 min (1,200 yd) Walk 2 min (200 yd) 2×	Off	Jog 8 min (1,200 yd) Walk 2 min (200 yd) 2×	Jog 8 min (1,200 yd) Walk 2 min (200 yd) 2×	Off	Jog 8 min (1,200 yd) Walk 2 min (200 yd) 2×	Jog 8 min (1,200 yd) Walk 2 min (200 yd) 2×
7	Jog 10 min (1,500 yd) Walk 2 min (200 yd) 2×	Jog 10 min (1,500 yd) Walk 2 min (200 yd) 2×	Off	Jog 10 min (1,500 yd) Walk 2 min (200 yd) 2×	Jog 10 min (1,500 yd) Walk 2 min (200 yd) 2×	Off	Jog 10 min (1,500 yd) Walk 2 min (200 yd) 2×
8	Jog 12 min (1,760 yd [1 mi]) Walk 2 min (200 yd) 2×	Off	Jog 12 min (1,760 yd [1 mi]) Walk 2 min (200 yd) 2×	Jog 12 min (1,760 yd [1 mi]) Walk 2 min (200 yd) 2×	Off	Jog 12 min (1,760 yd [1 mi]) Walk 2 min (200 yd) 2×	Jog 12 min (1,760 yd [1 mi]) Walk 2 min (200 yd) 2×

Walk briskly at an RPE of 11 or 12. Jog at an RPE of 13 to 15. Meters = yards × 0.91.
Reprinted by permission from Sharkey and Gaskill, 2007, p. 121, as adapted from President's Council on Physical Fitness and Sports, 1975.

INTERMEDIATE JOG–RUN PROGRAM

If you were already reasonably active, or if you've worked your way through the portions of the red, white, and blue programs that apply to you, then you're ready for the intermediate jog–run program (see the table beginning on page 80). This means you should be able to jog 1 mile (1.6 km) slowly and comfortably, rest 2 minutes, and then jog another mile. This kind of session consumes about 250 calories.

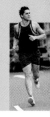

At this point, you're ready to progress in both intensity and duration. To determine intensity, you can use the rating of perceived exertion (see RPE numbers in parentheses in the table beginning on the following page). To start with, you'll jog 1 mile (1.6 km) in 12 minutes; by the time you finish this program, you may be able to complete 3 miles (4.8 km) or even more at a pace of 8 to 10 minutes per mile. Throughout this program, each week includes three phases:

RPE
6
7
8
9
10
11
12
13
14
15
16
17
18
19
20

➤ The basic workout

➤ Longer runs (overdistance)

➤ Shorter runs (underdistance)

If a given week's program seems too easy, move ahead; if it seems too hard, move back a week or two. On most days, the program calls for you to jog in intervals and walk to recover. For example, during the first week, you begin the Tuesday workout by slowly jogging 0.5 mile (0.8 km). You can start at 0.25 mile (0.4 km) if you need to. Then you try to jog 0.5 mile at a normal pace (for example, in 5 minutes 30 seconds), walk to recover, and repeat. Next, you jog 0.25 mile at the same pace (in our example, 2 minutes 45 seconds per quarter mile), walk to recover, and repeat three times. You then close the workout as you began it, by slowly jogging 0.5 mile. On Thursday, you jog 1 mile at a normal pace (in our example, 12 minutes), walk to recover, and repeat. Remember to warm up and cool down as part of every exercise session. You can read more about warm-up and stretching in chapter 6, pages 139 to 145. After you have warmed up with light activity to increase your body temperature, you might consider using some of the dynamic walking and jogging exercises found in chapter 7 (see page 161 for more on this).

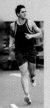

JOG–RUN PROGRAM

Intermediate Jog–Run Program

Week	Monday	Tuesday	Wednesday	Thursday	Friday	Saturday or Sunday
1	1 mile jog (13 or 14) Walk 3–4 min 2×	1/2 mile slow jog (13) 2× 1/2 mile (14) 4× 1/4 mile (15) 1/2 mile slow jog (13)	2 mile slow jog (13)	1 mile jog (13 or 14) Walk 3–4 min 2×	1/2 mile slow jog (13) 2× 1/2 mile (14) 4× 1/4 mile (15) 1/2 mile slow jog (13)	2 mile slow jog (13)
2	1 mile jog (13 or 14) Walk 3–4 min 2× Your mile time should be about 10–15 sec faster than in week 1.	1/2 mile slow jog (13) 1/2 mile (14) 2× 1/4 mile (16) 2× 1/4 mile (15) 4× 220 yd (15 or 16) 1/2 mile slow jog (13)	Brisk walk 30–60 min (12)	1 mile jog (13 or 14) Walk 3–4 min 2× Your mile time should be about 10–15 sec faster than in week 1.	1/2 mile slow jog (13) 1/2 mile (14) 2× 1/4 mile (16) 2× 1/4 mile (15) 4× 220 yd (15 or 16) 1/2 mile slow jog (13)	2 1/4 mile slow jog (13) or Brisk walk 30–60 min (12)
3	1 mile jog (13 or 14) Walk 3–4 min 2× Your mile time should be about 5–10 sec faster than in week 2.	1/2 mile slow jog (13) 1/2 mile (15) 4× 1/4 mile (14) 4× 220 yd (16) 4× 100 yd (16) 1/2 mile slow jog (13)	2 1/2 mile slow jog (13) or Brisk walk 30–60 min (12)	1 mile jog (13 or 14) Walk 3–4 min 2× Your mile time should be about 5–10 sec faster than in week 2.	1/2 mile slow jog (13) 1/2 mile (15) 4× 1/4 mile (14) 4× 220 yd (16) 4× 100 yd (16) 1/2 mile slow jog (13)	2 1/2 mile slow jog (13) or Brisk walk 30–60 min (12)

Values in parentheses match ratings of perceived exertion. See pp. 46-47.

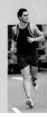

Week	Monday	Tuesday	Wednesday	Thursday	Friday	Saturday or Sunday
4	1 mile jog (13–15) Walk 3–4 min 2× Your mile time should be about 5–10 sec faster than in week 3.	1/2 mile slow jog (13) 2× 1/2 mile (14) 4× 1/4 mile (16) 4× 220 yd (15) 1/2 mile slow jog (13)	2 3/4 mile slow jog (13) or Brisk walk 45–70 min (12)	1 mile jog (13–15) Walk 3–4 min 2× Your mile time should be about 5–10 sec faster than in week 3.	1/2 mile slow jog (13) 2× 1/2 mile (14) 4× 1/4 mile (16) 4× 220 yd (15) 1/2 mile slow jog (13)	2 3/4 mile slow jog (13) or Brisk walk 45–70 min (12)
5 Easier week	1 mile jog (13 or 14) Walk 3–5 min 2× Your mile time should be about the same as in the previous week.	Off	3 mile slow jog (13)	1 mile jog (13 or 14) Walk 3–5 min 2× Your mile time should be about the same as in the previous week.	1/2 mile slow jog (13) 1/2 mile (15) 4× 1/4 mile (16) 4× 220 yd (15) 4× 100 yd (14) 1/2 mile slow jog (13)	Brisk walk 45–70 min (11 or 12)
6 Harder week	1 1/2 mile jog (13–15) Maintain same pace as in weeks 4 and 5.	1/2 mile slow jog (13) 2× 1/2 mile (15) 4× 1/4 mile (16) 4× 220 yd (15) 4× 100 yd (16) 1/2 mile slow jog (13)	3 mile slow jog (13), increasing the pace the last 5–8 min (15)	1 1/2 mile jog (13–15) Walk 5–6 min 2× Maintain same pace as in weeks 4 and 5.	1/2 mile slow jog (13) 2× 1/2 mile (15) 4× 1/4 mile (16) 4× 220 yd (15) 4× 100 yd (16) 1/2 mile slow jog (13)	4 mile slow jog (13)

(continued)

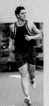

JOG–RUN PROGRAM *(continued)*

Week	Monday	Tuesday	Wednesday	Thursday	Friday	Saturday or Sunday
7 Medium week	1 mile jog (14 or 15) Walk 3–5 min 2× Your mile time should be about 5–10 sec faster than in the previous 3 weeks.	1/2 mile slow jog (13) 2× 1/2 mile (15) 3× 1/4 mile (16) 3× 220 yd (15) 1/2 mile slow jog (13)	3 mile slow jog (13)	1 mile jog (14 or 15) Walk 3–5 min 2× Your mile time should be about 5–10 sec faster than in the previous 3 weeks.	1/2 mile slow jog (13) 2× 1/2 mile (15) 3× 1/4 mile (16) 3× 220 yd (15) 1/2 mile slow jog (13)	3 1/2 mile slow jog (13)
8 Hard week	1 mile jog (15) Walk 3–5 min 1 mile jog (14) 2× The first mile of each set should be slightly faster than in week 7.	1/2 mile slow jog (13) 2× 1/2 mile (15) 4× 1/4 mile (16) 4× 220 yd (16) 4× 100 yd (15) 1/2 mile slow jog (13)	3 1/2 mile slow jog (13)	1 mile jog (15) Walk 3–5 min 1 mile jog (14) 2× The first mile of each set should be slightly faster than in week 7.	Off	5 mile slow jog (13)
9 Easy week	1 mile jog (14) Walk 3–5 min 2× Your mile time should be about the same as in week 7.	1/2 mile slow jog (13) 2× 1/2 mile (15) 3× 1/4 mile (15) 4× 220 yd (16) 4× 50 yd (16) 1/2 mile slow jog (13)	3 mile slow jog (13)	1 mile jog (14) Walk 3–5 min 2× Your mile time should be about the same as in week 7.	1/2 mile slow jog (13) 2× 1/2 mile (15) 3× 1/4 mile (15) 4× 220 yd (16) 4× 50 yd (16) 1/2 mile slow jog (13)	4 mile slow jog (13)

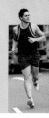

Week	Monday	Tuesday	Wednesday	Thursday	Friday	Saturday or Sunday
10 Harder week	1 1/2 mile jog (13–15) Walk 4–6 min 2× Maintain same pace as in week 9.	1/2 mile slow jog (13) 2× 1/2 mile (16) 3× 1/4 mile (14) 4× 220 yd (17) 1/2 mile slow jog (13)	4 mile slow jog (13), increasing the pace the last 8–10 min (15)	1 1/2 mile jog (13–15) Walk 4–6 min 2× Maintain same pace as in week 9.	1/2 mile slow jog (13) 2× 1/2 mile (16) 3× 1/4 mile (14) 4× 220 yd (17) 1/2 mile slow jog (13)	6 mile slow jog (13)
11 Medium week	1 mile jog (14 or 15) Walk 3–5 min 3× Your mile time should be about 10 sec faster than in week 10.	1/2 mile slow jog (13) 4× 1/2 mile (15) 4× 1/4 mile (16) 2× 220 yd (17) 1/2 mile slow jog (13)	4 mile slow jog (13)	Off	1/2 mile slow jog (13) 4× 1/2 mile (15) 4× 1/4 mile (16) 2× 220 yd (17) 1/2 mile slow jog (13)	5 mile slow jog (13)
12 Hard week	1 1/2 mile jog (13–15) Walk 4–6 min 2× Maintain same pace as in week 11.	1/2 mile slow jog (13) 5× 1/2 mile (16) 4× 1/4 mile (15) 4× 220 yd (16) 2× 100 yd (17) 1/2 mile slow jog (13)	4 mile easy jog (13), increasing the pace the last 8–10 min (15)	1 1/2 mile jog (13–15) Walk 4–6 min 2× Maintain same pace as in week 11.	1/2 mile slow jog (13) 5× 1/2 mile (16) 4× 1/4 mile (15) 4× 220 yd (16) 2× 100 yd (17) 1/2 mile slow jog (13)	6 mile slow jog (13 or 14)

Values in parentheses match ratings of perceived exertion. See pp. 46-47. Meters = yards × 0.91. Kilometers = miles × 1.61.

Reprinted by permission from Sharkey and Gaskill, 2007, pp. 123-124.

Advanced Aerobic Fitness Training

This section provides suggestions for advanced training. Remember, however, that there is no single best way to train. If you enjoy under-distance—going short and fast—then by all means, do it. If, instead, you enjoy training at lower intensity over a longer distance (overdistance), then take that approach. This latter approach can still give you an optimal training stimulus if you simply increase your pace as you approach the end of your workout. You may also enjoy the fact that, because the speed work is limited to a short span near the end of your effort, the discomfort is brief. I provide programs for cycling and swimming, but you can incorporate many other types of aerobic activities into your program. If you have the inclination and the equipment, you might try paddling or rowing, cross-country skiing, or even competitive sports such as basketball and soccer.

The following suggestions can help you make your training sessions productive and safe:

➤ Always warm up before your session; do so by walking slowly, marching briskly, or jogging in place for a few minutes.

➤ Stretch *after* warming up; see chapter 6 for specific information about stretching.

➤ Vary the distance, intensity, and location of your training (e.g., long or short, fast or slow, hilly or flat).

➤ Set goals for distance, but don't become a slave to your goals; increase distance only if you enjoy it.

➤ Use an alternate-day schedule, or, if you like, train 6 days per week.

➤ Try doing one long run on either Saturday or Sunday (don't go farther than one-third of your total weekly distance).

➤ If the longer run seems too hard, try two shorter runs—for example, two 5-mile (8 km) runs instead of one 10-mile (16 km) run.

➤ Build recovery time into your plan by including an easier week every 3 or 4 weeks.

➤ If you like, keep records of your training (dates, distances, and comments about the run, the location, and how you felt). You'll be surprised! You might also note your wake-up heart rate and body weight. In addition, check your performance over a measured distance at least once—or several times, if you like—a year in order to formally track your progress (you can use a local road race for this purpose or perform the 1.5-mile [2.4 km] run test discussed on page 26 in chapter 2).

➤ Don't train with a stopwatch because that will make you focus too much on intensity, but do wear a watch so you can track how long you've trained.

➤ After training, *always* cool down. You can do this simply by slowing your pace for the last few minutes so that your body's systems can recover to their resting levels.

The cycling and swimming programs combine the training concepts outlined earlier to provide safe, effective, and engaging approaches to fitness and performance. You can use these programs to improve your fitness and then switch to a maintenance program once you reach your targeted fitness level. It is not necessary to improve your fitness to a high level unless you are training for a particular event; fortunately, the health benefits are available to you if you simply remain active.

CYCLING PROGRAM

In this program, you guide your progress by means of a weekly training menu (see the table below):

Monday	**Easy distance**—ride at a comfortable pace (RPE = 13).
Tuesday	**Pace**—cycle at a brisk pace (RPE = 15).
Wednesday	**Hills**—build stamina (RPE = 14).
Thursday	**Intervals**—push harder for brief intervals (RPE = 15); after 4 weeks, increase to RPE = 16.
Friday	**Overdistance**—go easy to develop endurance (RPE = 11).
Saturday	**Variety**—try a different activity (e.g., tennis or hiking) or ride a trail.
Sunday	**Rest**—or try a light activity (e.g., gardening or walking).

After 8 weeks, step out on your own a bit and design a program to suit your particular needs and interests. In addition to using elements from this plan, you might integrate other approaches that appeal to you. You might even plan a long cycling trip with friends and schedule training rides together.

Cycling Program

	WEEK							
	1	2	3	4	5	6	7	8
Monday	30 min	40 min	50 min	40 min	50 min	60 min	70 min	60 min
Tuesday	2 × 10 min	2 × 15 min	2 × 20 min	3 × 10 min	3 × 15 min	3 × 20 min	4 × 10 min	4 × 15 min
Wednesday	15 min	20 min	25 min	20 min	2 × 15 min	2 × 20 min	2 × 25 min	3 × 20 min
Thursday	3 × 3 min	3 × 4 min	3 × 5 min	3 × 6 min	4 × 3 min	4 × 4 min	4 × 5 min	5 × 5 min
Friday	60 min	70 min	80 min	75 min	90 min	100 min	110 min	120 min

Always wear a helmet; ride easy to warm up.

Pace: Ride for 10 minutes, relax and recover, and then ride another set. Hills: Include some standing but try to keep RPE at 14. Intervals: Ride one, cycle easy to recover, and then ride the next. Overdistance: Ride easy; stop for rest and fluids every 30 minutes.

Reprinted by permission from Sharkey and Gaskill, 2007, p. 126.

This program requires that you have a certain amount of swimming skill (see the table below). If it seems too difficult at this point, you can scale it down and take lessons in order to develop your skill and efficiency. Here is the weekly training menu:

Monday	**Easy distance**—go easy at a comfortable pace (RPE = 12).
Tuesday	**Pace**—swim at a firm pace (RPE = 15).
Wednesday	**Arms and legs**—swim with arms only and then legs only (RPE = 13).
Thursday	**Intervals**—swim harder for brief intervals (RPE = 15); after 4 weeks, increase to RPE = 16.
Friday	**Overdistance**—relax on a longer swim (RPE = 11).
Saturday	**Variety**—try a different activity or a water game (e.g., water polo).
Sunday	**Rest**—or try a light activity (e.g., gardening or walking).

Swimming Program

	WEEK							
	1	2	3	4	5	6	7	8
Monday	15 min	20 min	25 min	20 min	25 min	30 min	35 min	30 min
Tuesday	2 × 5 min	2 × 6 min	2 × 7 min	2 × 8 min	3 × 6 min	3 × 7 min	3 × 8 min	4 × 5 min
Wednesday	5 min arms, then 5 min legs	6 min arms, then 6 min legs	7 min arms, then 7 min legs	8 min arms, then 8 min legs	9 min arms, then 9 min legs	10 min arms, then 10 min legs	11 min arms, then 11 min legs	12 min arms, then 12 min legs
Thursday	3 × 3 min	3 × 4 min	3 × 5 min	3 × 4 min	4 × 3 min	4 × 4 min	4 × 5 min	5 × 4 min
Friday	25 min	30 min	35 min	40 min	35 min	40 min	45 min	50 min

Use good goggles. Warm up well on Tuesday, Wednesday, and Thursday; swim easy laps after these workouts.

Pace and intervals: Swim slowly or walk in the water to recover between sets. Arms and legs: Use a kickboard or flotation device for support.

Reprinted by permission from Sharkey and Gaskill, 2007, p. 126.

Once you have completed all 8 weeks, you might enjoy designing your own program consisting of the types of training that appeal most to you. You might even decide to train for a triathlon like Sister Madonna Buder!

Is Cross-Training Effective?

Does running, swimming, or cycling enhance performance in another sport? The bad news is that cross-training doesn't work that way; in order to improve performance, training must be specific. The good news, however, is that it still makes sense to vary your training. Here are several reasons:

- To train for a multisport event like the triathlon
- To add variety to your training and relieve the potential boredom of constant running, swimming, or cycling
- And, most important, to reduce the impact and risk of overuse injury associated with repetitive activities such as running

During the summer, I run and mountain-bike; for diversion, I also do hiking, paddling, swimming, and golf. My winter activities include cross-country and downhill skiing, snowshoeing, and some running, and my winter diversions involve backcountry ski trips. I also do one or two weight-lifting sessions during most weeks throughout the year in order to maintain muscular fitness and improve or maintain performance. Fall and spring serve as transition periods for me, and they are enhanced by new activities and new locales. I recommend trying more than one mode of exercise to burn calories and train some muscles while resting others. You'll like it!

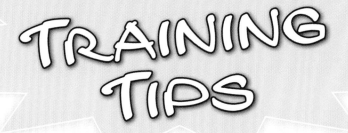

TRAINING TIPS

I have written these tips with walking and running in mind because they provide a great training stimulus for the time and money you put into them. You can do these activities at any time and in almost any weather, and you can easily control both intensity and duration. The needed equipment is relatively inexpensive; it is also light and easily packed on vacation or business trips. Furthermore, you can do these activities either alone or in a group, and you can continue doing them throughout your life. Thus, walking and running offer you two excellent ways to achieve and maintain the health benefits associated with aerobic fitness. Of course, if you choose other modes of activity, that is all right! Just apply these tips to your chosen physical activity.

FitFact

Cross-training reduces your risk of overuse injuries, and its inherent variety eliminates the boredom of unrelenting training.

What to Wear

Your enjoyment of walking and running depends as much as anything on your shoes, so, unless you know something about the product, this is not the time to buy sale shoes at a discount outlet. Instead, seek advice from a knowledgeable salesperson at a reputable sporting goods dealer. Avoid shoes built for competition; a training shoe will serve you best.

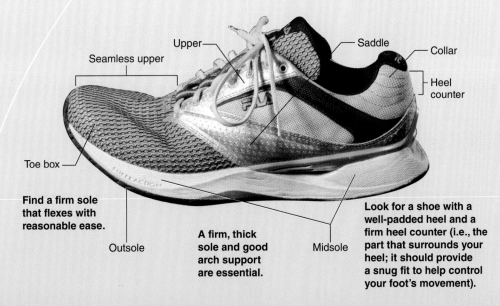

Seamless upper · Upper · Saddle · Collar · Heel counter · Toe box

Find a firm sole that flexes with reasonable ease.

Outsole

A firm, thick sole and good arch support are essential.

Midsole

Look for a shoe with a well-padded heel and a firm heel counter (i.e., the part that surrounds your heel; it should provide a snug fit to help control your foot's movement).

If you find that blisters pose a problem for you, try wearing tube socks, wearing a thin sock under a heavier one, or applying a balm to lubricate problem spots (try Bag Balm from a livestock outlet—yes, it was created for cow udders, but it works great for athletes as well!).

You don't need to wear fancy clothing to enjoy walking and jogging. In warmer weather, nylon or cotton shorts and a T-shirt will do the job. In colder environments, you can rely on a jogging suit until the thermometer dips below 20 degrees Fahrenheit (minus 7 degrees Celsius); some runners prefer tights. In any case, remember that lighter layers work better than one heavy garment. This way, you can peel off a layer as you heat up. As you find it necessary in cold weather, add gloves and a knit cap. In windy weather, use a thin windbreaker to reduce heat loss from wind chill. When it is *really* cold, try wearing tights under wind pants. Many runners continue to venture forth even in subzero temperatures, and you can do this safely if you wear proper clothing, warm up, and remain vigilant for signs of frostbite (such as tingling, burning, and eventually numbing of the affected extremities). For longer winter outings, I use polypropylene underwear that wicks perspiration away from my skin and thus prevents rapid cooling, which can lead to hypothermia. Add a pile vest and a windbreaker on top, and you're good to go.

lighter layers work better

Technique

If you are running faster than a jog, lean forward slightly, lift your knees higher, push off more quickly and forcefully, and use more arm action.

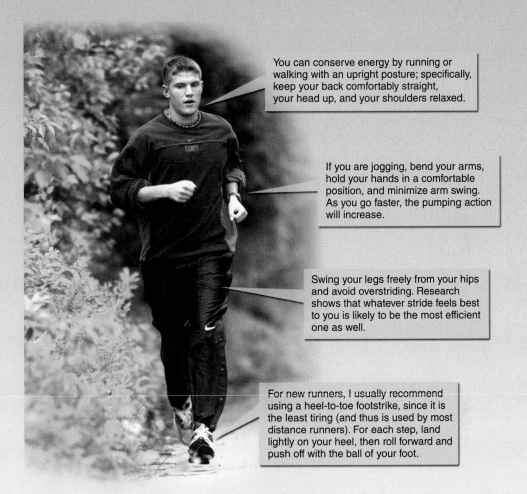

You can conserve energy by running or walking with an upright posture; specifically, keep your back comfortably straight, your head up, and your shoulders relaxed.

If you are jogging, bend your arms, hold your hands in a comfortable position, and minimize arm swing. As you go faster, the pumping action will increase.

Swing your legs freely from your hips and avoid overstriding. Research shows that whatever stride feels best to you is likely to be the most efficient one as well.

For new runners, I usually recommend using a heel-to-toe footstrike, since it is the least tiring (and thus is used by most distance runners). For each step, land lightly on your heel, then roll forward and push off with the ball of your foot.

Time of Day

Exercise at whatever time works best for you. Some folks like to get it done before breakfast. Others prefer to run during the lunch hour; in fact, if you have a problem at work, you'll often come back from an exercise session with the solution. Still others get their fix right after work, and a few night owls prefer to brave the dark (a run and a shower help them sleep). Take care, however, to avoid vigorous exercise during the first hour or two after a meal, when your digestive system requires considerable blood supply. Activities that do not involve bouncing, such as walking, cycling, and cross-country skiing, are safe to do shortly after eating. Unless you need time alone, consider training with a partner who shares your ability level, interests, and goals; pairing up in this way can help you stick to your exercise schedule.

Where to Train

When you begin training, avoid exercising on hard surfaces that could bruise your feet. There are, after all, plenty of other options, and the variety will help you maintain interest and enjoyment. You might walk or run in a park, on a playing field, on a golf course when allowed, or on a running track. After a few weeks, you'll be ready to try back roads or trails in your area. When the weather forces you indoors, try a mall, YMCA, or school gym; another option is to default to an exercise supplement that you can do at home, such as jumping rope or using a stationary bike or other indoor exercise equipment.

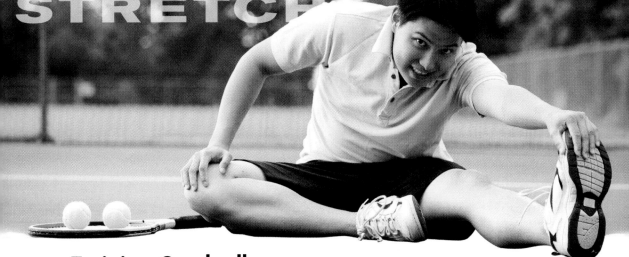

Training Gradually

When a previously inactive person begins training, problems sometimes arise, but you can steer clear of this obstacle if you make haste slowly. You got out of shape over a period of years, and you won't turn things around in a day or a week. Instead, plan to make gradual progress; in the beginning, too little may be better than too much. If you stick with a good plan, you'll find after several weeks that your body has begun adjusting to the demands of vigorous effort and therefore that you're ready to increase the intensity or duration of your workout. You can further smooth your path to fitness by taking time to warm up and stretch before each exercise session—and to cool down after your workout. Doing so makes you less likely to suffer the nagging physical problems that often plague less patient exercisers. See chapter 9 for information about common activity problems and how to treat them.

Keys to Aerobic Programs

➤ To figure out where to start, take the walk test or the walk–jog test.
➤ Design a program to fit the rhythm of your life.
➤ Start easy and make haste slowly.
➤ Increase duration, then frequency, and finally intensity.
➤ Do advanced training if it suits your goals.
➤ Do cross-training to reduce stress and strain and to expand your horizons.

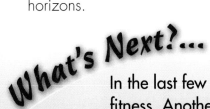

In the last few chapters, we have considered aerobic fitness. Another part of fitness is muscular fitness, which involves building muscular strength and endurance. In chapter 5, you'll learn how your muscles work—and how they change with muscular fitness training.

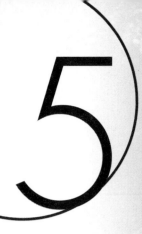

5

Understanding Muscular Fitness

Strength
and
Endurance

Power waits upon him
who earns it.

~ John Burroughs

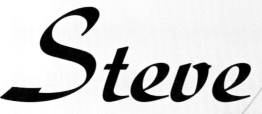

Steve

was comfortable in his office job.

But when the economy turned sour, his company was hit hard. Steve was laid off, and he struggled to find work. With a wife and two children, he couldn't go without a paycheck, so he put his engineering skills to work as a handyman and began doing minor construction and remodeling work. After his first week of experimenting with this new line of work, Steve realized that he was very out of shape in terms of his muscle strength and endurance. If he was going to continue doing construction work, he would have to get fit.

...he needed to gain strength

He needed to be able to stay strong throughout the day, and he also knew that he needed to gain strength so that he wouldn't suffer an injury doing something that he wasn't ready for. Given his financial situation, however, Steve couldn't afford to join a health club, so what was he to do? He found a few quick tips on the Web, got advice from a knowledgeable friend, and then read a reputable book on strength training. He devised a program that focused first on building strength through resistance training three times a week. He started with light weights and built up gradually to doing 8 to 10 reps of each exercise with fairly heavy weights. After a few weeks, he transitioned to working on his muscular endurance by using slightly lighter weights but doing more repetitions. Steve quickly saw a difference in his performance on the job. Now enjoying the stamina to last through the day—and the ability to do heavy work without fear of injury—he soon felt comfortable in his new line of work.

Use It or Lose It

You probably know that muscular fitness is important in many sports and in some forms of work, such as construction and firefighting. But did you know that muscular fitness can also contribute substantially to your health and quality of life?

➤ Training for muscular fitness increases your muscle mass, which in turn burns fat.

➤ Exercises that improve your muscular fitness help you avoid osteoporosis, the crippling bone demineralization that afflicts many older people.

➤ If you achieve and maintain muscular fitness, you may be able to avoid low-back problems and repetitive strain injuries.

➤ Good muscular fitness maximizes your chance for independence and mobility in your later years.

Muscular fitness consists of three basics: strength, muscular endurance, and flexibility. Other elements include power, agility, balance, and coordination. As with most physiologic capabilities, you either use muscular fitness or you lose it. The cold, hard fact is that your strength, endurance, flexibility, power, agility, and balance will all decline with age. The good news is that you can reduce this rate of decline by being active. Research shows that we can build strength even in our 90s! But don't let this fool you into waiting—the pleasures and rewards of muscular fitness are worth pursuing as soon as possible. Begin now and you will soon notice that you are getting things done more easily, that your tummy is flatter and your muscles firmer, and that you feel better about yourself and your life.

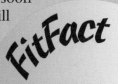

FitFact

If you train your muscles, they will be able to burn more fat.

Aerobic and muscular fitness both contribute to health, but they do so in different ways and at different times.

20s

If you're young, you might use muscular fitness to improve your performance in a sport or to look good in a bathing suit.

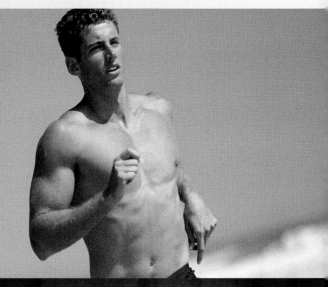

40s

If you're middle-aged, you might be more interested in exercising for abdominal tone and flexibility in order to prevent or minimize low-back problems.

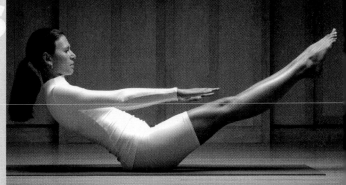

60s

If you're older, you might do activities that develop strength and muscular endurance to help you retain bone density and stay active, able to perform the basics of daily living, and thus remain independent.

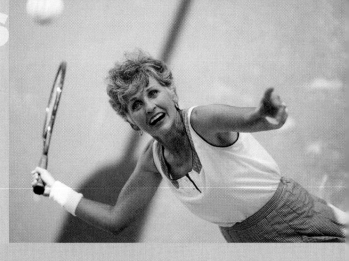

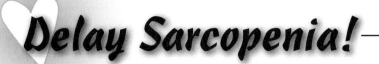

Delay Sarcopenia!

Strength declines rather slowly with age until your 40s or 50s, when the rate of decline increases. This loss of muscle has been called sarcopenia, or vanishing flesh, and it contributes to frailty in elderly persons by reducing their strength and thus increasing their risk of falls and fractures. Sarcopenia results from the loss of muscle fibers and from fiber atrophy, due to lack of use, and from a decrease in muscle-building hormones (e.g., testosterone). If you use your strength regularly, however, you will retain muscle function much longer. Furthermore, research shows that very elderly men and women (average age 87 years) can counter muscle weakness and frailty with muscular fitness training (Fiatarone et al. 1994).

How Do Muscles Work?

Each of your muscles contains thousands of spaghetti-like fibers that range in length from half an inch to 12 inches (about 1 to 30 cm). Your muscles shorten to produce movement when contractile proteins creep or slide along each other. This creeping is brought about when tiny cross-bridges, extending from thicker to thinner filaments, reach out, make contact, and pull like oars. In any one location, this movement is barely perceptible, but when it is all added together, it produces movement along the length of the fiber, and your body moves visibly. Because your muscles are attached to bony lever systems throughout your body, this rather modest muscle shortening is multiplied to produce the bodily movements with which you are familiar.

Human muscle is composed of two fiber types—fast-twitch and slow-twitch. All the fibers in a given motor unit are of the same type (either fast- or slow-twitch), but each muscle has a combination of the two; it's just a matter of which type is more prevalent and which is called on to produce a movement. Your fast-twitch fibers are larger and have fewer capillaries than your slow-twitch fibers; they contract fast and fatigue fast and thus seem best suited to short, intense effort. In contrast, your slow-twitch fibers enjoy rich capillary support and are well supplied with the metabolism required for endurance activities; they are slower to contract and slower to fatigue. When your nervous system commands a motor unit to contract, all the fibers respond together, and the characteristics of your muscle fibers seem to be dictated by the way your nervous system uses them (i.e., for short, intense effort or for long-duration effort; see the table on page 102).

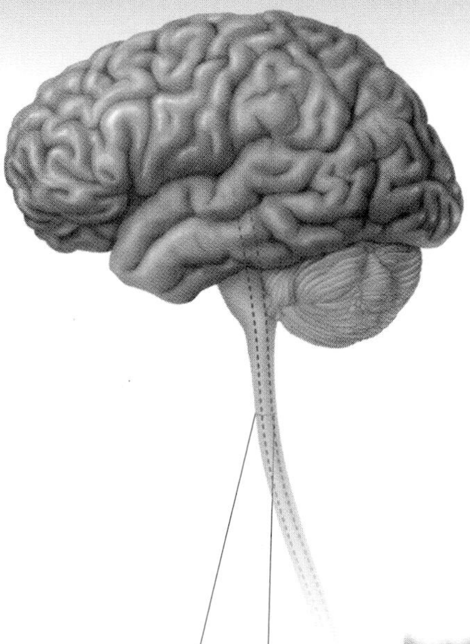

Muscle fibers contract at the command of the brain (motor cortex) and the motor nerve. Because each motor nerve branches many times, the typical neuron activates an average of 150 individual muscle fibers simultaneously. The motor nerve and the muscle fibers it commands make up a motor unit.

Every muscle contains thousands of muscle fibers. Inside the muscle fibers are thick and thin filaments, which are made up of proteins.

Tiny cross-bridges extend from the thicker to the thinner filaments. The cross-bridges reach out, make contact, and pull like oars. This causes the muscle to shorten, which produces movement.

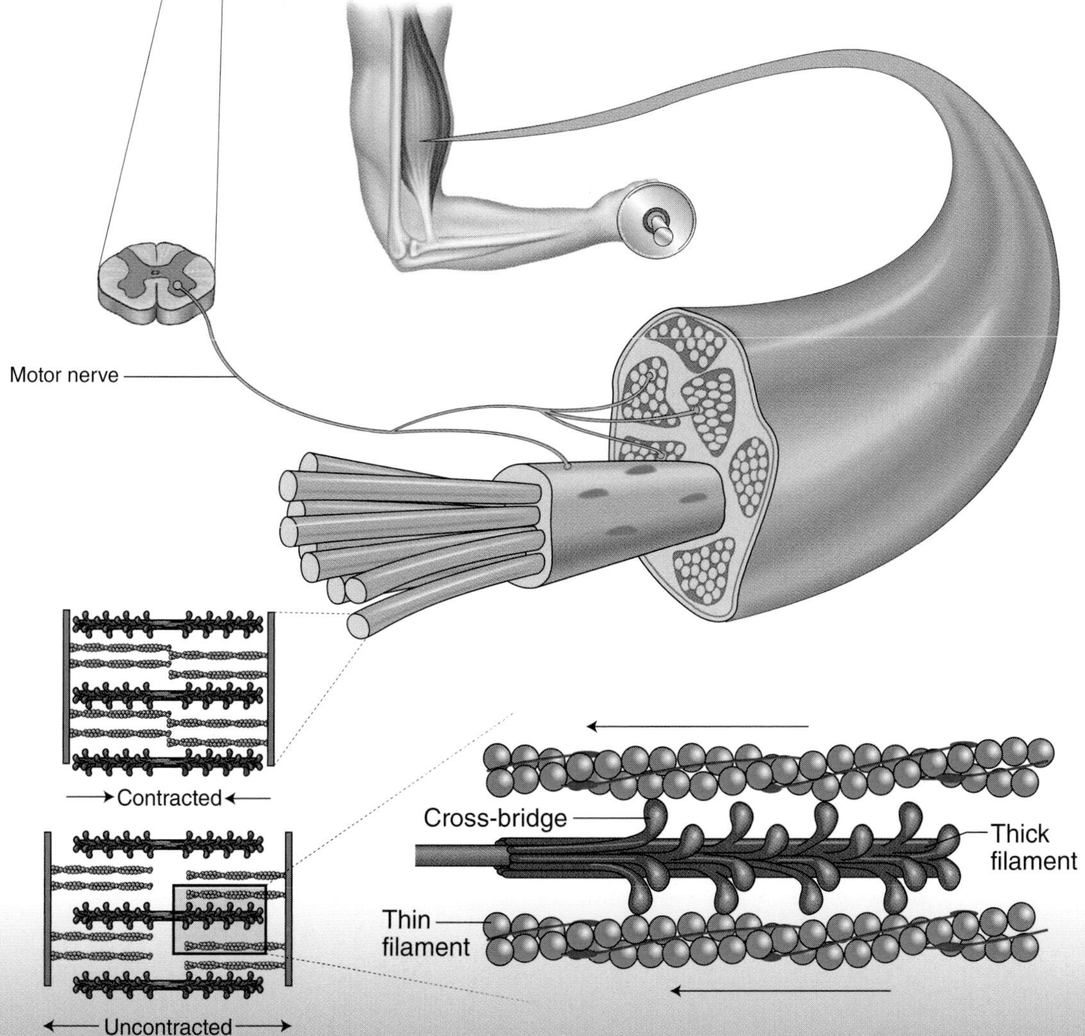

Motor nerve

Contracted

Uncontracted

Cross-bridge

Thick filament

Thin filament

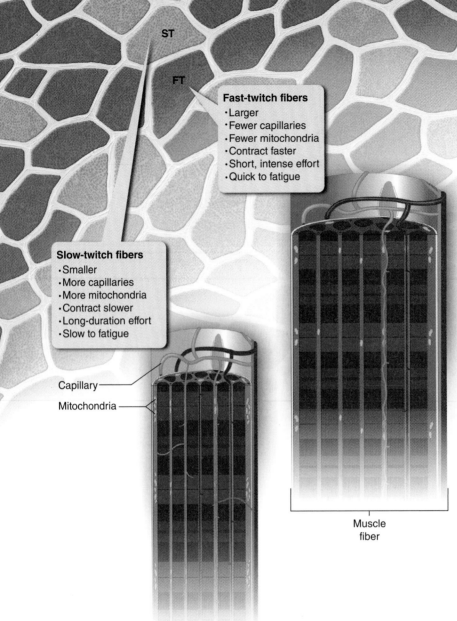

ST

FT

Fast-twitch fibers
- Larger
- Fewer capillaries
- Fewer mitochondria
- Contract faster
- Short, intense effort
- Quick to fatigue

Slow-twitch fibers
- Smaller
- More capillaries
- More mitochondria
- Contract slower
- Long-duration effort
- Slow to fatigue

Capillary

Mitochondria

Muscle
fiber

Characteristics of Muscle Fibers

Characteristics	Slow-twitch	Fast-twitch
Average fiber percentage	50	50
Speed of contraction	Slow	Fast
Size	Smaller	Larger
Fatigability	Fatigue-resistant	More easily fatigued
Aerobic capacity	High	Medium to low

Now that you know how your muscles work, let's look at those three primary components of muscular fitness—strength, muscular endurance, and flexibility—and consider how training changes your muscles. These three components are considered primary because they are the ones most related to health. In addition, muscular fitness, along with other movement experiences, can improve your balance and agility. Other components—power, speed, and coordination—gain importance if you want to improve performance in a sport or activity.

Strength

Strength comes from lifting heavy loads. It is defined as the maximal force that you can exert in a single *voluntary* contraction, meaning that you are doing it on purpose. This amount of force is also called a 1-repetition maximum, or 1RM. It's the most that you can lift or pull or push one time. Strength is important in certain occupations (e.g., construction, a nurse moving a patient), in some sports (e.g., mountain biking in hills), and, perhaps surprisingly, for people over 60 years of age (for activities of daily living).

We need strength throughout our lives in order to handle emergencies, minimize injury, and live fully and independently. You use strength, for example, every time you change a flat tire, dig a hole in the garden, or lift and carry a child or a bag of groceries. If, however, your strength and muscular fitness are low, you are likely to be less active, thereby hastening your natural loss of strength and initiating a vicious cycle that will reduce your quality of life and independence and might eventually land you in a nursing home. But take heart! You can begin taking steps today to reverse this cycle and enable yourself to live independently well into your 80s.

Strength training improves both slow- and fast-twitch muscle fibers, but the effects are most noticeable in fast-twitch fibers. Training increases the contractile proteins that are essential to muscle contraction and to developing stronger connective tissue (such as membranes, ligaments, and tendons).

Most of us do not use our full strength. In fact, we unknowingly *inhibit* the full expression of our strength. Both your brain and inhibitory receptors in your muscles hold back in a sense and thus prevent you from using your full measure of strength. Strength training, however, reduces these inhibitions and thus allows you to use your available strength more fully. When you strengthen a muscle through training, the early changes hinge on reducing the inhibitions in your brain and muscle receptors so that they allow your muscle to express more of its strength. As you continue training, increased strength derives from changes in the muscle fibers themselves.

If you want to live as independently as possible and enjoy your life to the fullest, it is important that you maintain adequate strength throughout your life. If you're older, you need strength to get out of a chair, to walk, to climb stairs, and to carry groceries. If you want to travel, you'll need to be able to handle the rigors it entails (e.g., moving your luggage through airports), which means you'll need even more strength. Thus, if you want to enjoy your retirement, you should get involved in strength training and other forms of muscular fitness training now.

Muscular Endurance

Muscular endurance is the ability to repeat muscular contractions for a period of time. For example, you need muscular endurance in order to load boxes onto a moving truck. You also need it if you are going to pedal a bicycle for an hour or hammer nails for 30 minutes. And you need it in order to swim or to walk 18 holes of golf.

Once you have gained the strength to perform a repetitive task, you can further improve your performance by developing muscular endurance—the ability to persist. Since persistence is often required in sport, work, and life, your success depends in no small part on your muscular endurance. We develop skill through repeated action, which of course requires endurance; you need muscular endurance in order to practice, train, and perform. Contrary to common perception, muscular endurance and strength are not highly related.

You achieve muscular endurance by repeatedly contracting your muscle fibers. To do this, you need a continuous supply of energy, and the muscle fibers that possess endurance capabilities (i.e., your slow-twitch fibers) fit the bill. Notice the cycle: When you do repetitive contractions, you enhance the aerobic enzymes, mitochondria (organelles in your muscle cells that help generate energy), and fuels that are needed to do repetitive contractions.

FitFact

If you want to lift a heavy object one time, you need *strength*. If you want to lift a moderately heavy box many times, you're looking for *muscular endurance*.

105

How Does Training Change Your Muscles?

Each type of training stimulates transcription of different genes within the DNA of the muscle cell nuclei.

Transcription of each gene produces a unique messenger RNA (mRNA) which is translated into a chain of amino acids with the help of ribosomes.

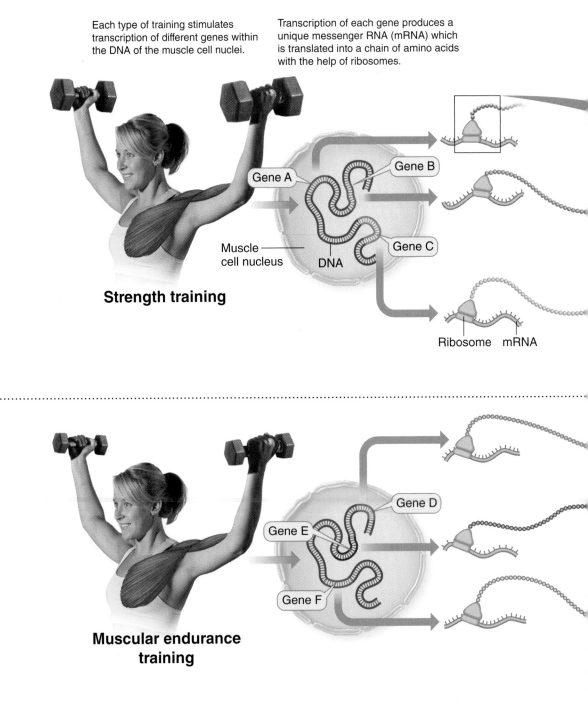

Strength training

Gene A

Gene B

Gene C

Muscle cell nucleus

DNA

Ribosome mRNA

Gene D

Gene E

Gene F

Muscular endurance training

Ribosomes translate each mRNA by recruiting transfer RNA molecules (tRNAs). Each tRNA brings with it an amino acid matching a specific code in the mRNA. The tRNA adds its amino acid to the chain of amino acids and then moves on.

The ribosome strings together the amino acids into a polypeptide chain. The sequence of amino acids in this chain determines how the chain will fold, and which protein will be formed from it.

— Growing chain of amino acids (polypeptide chain)

— Amino acid

— tRNA

Polypeptide encoded in Gene A is used to increase protein synthesis capacity, which helps repair and build muscle tissue.

Polypeptide encoded in Gene B is used to build more contractile proteins.

Polypeptide encoded in Gene C is used to toughen and thicken connective tissue.

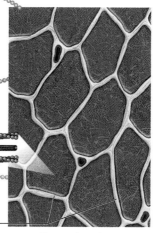

Strength-trained muscle cross-section

Polypeptide encoded in Gene D is used to build more aerobic enzymes.

Polypeptide encoded in Gene E is used in the conversion of type IIx to type IIa fibers, which have more mitochondria.

Polypeptide encoded in Gene F is used to build more capillaries.

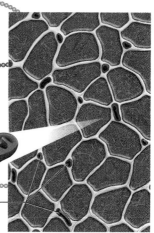

Muscular endurance–trained muscle cross-section

Muscular Versus Aerobic Endurance

Muscular endurance is different from aerobic endurance. A pianist or meat cutter, for instance, develops considerable endurance in small muscles such as finger flexors, but this has no noticeable effect on his or her heart or respiratory system. In fact, my barber has great endurance in the muscles of his fingers, but his aerobic fitness is poor. *Muscular* endurance resides in the ability of muscle fibers to extract energy from fat and carbohydrate, thereby allowing prolonged activity.

Just how does training generate changes in your muscles? The answer hinges in part on what you do to train. Your muscles respond specifically to the type of training you do. More precisely, training signals cell nuclei to make messenger RNA (mRNA), which is then sent into your muscle fiber to order the production of specific protein:

➤ Contractile protein for strength training
➤ Aerobic enzyme protein for endurance training

After it is formed, the mRNA's message is received by structures called ribosomes, which then produce the specific protein needed to adapt to the specific training stimulus. This process is enabled by another RNA (transfer RNA, or tRNA), which gathers amino acids and delivers them to the ribosome, where they are used to construct the desired protein. To benefit from training, then, you need to consume sufficient protein to provide these amino acid building blocks.

You improve your strength by applying sufficient overload (*tension*) to your targeted muscle fiber and its contractile proteins. To do so, you must move a load or weight that requires more than two-thirds of your muscle's maximal force. Think about it: If you lift a lightweight box, your muscles are of course working, but they do not gain strength because you are not making them work harder than usual. Thus, if you do contractions with less than two-thirds of your muscle's maximal force, you won't gain much strength. You will, however, gain muscular endurance. The number of repetitions is also important. Imagine now that you have to lift that lightweight box 20 times. You still won't gain much strength, but because your muscles might not be used to lifting that much weight 20 times in succession, you will gain muscular endurance from doing so. In the final analysis, as long as you exert enough tension for enough repetitions, you will benefit from doing any form of resistance training. Your individual progress will depend on your training level, the nutrition you take in, and your genetic endowment.

Results Are Specific!

As with aerobic endurance training, then, the principle of specificity applies here. Your muscles adapt according to the particular type of overload training you give them. Your muscles adapt to *strength* training by growing due to increases in their contractile proteins and the development of tougher connective tissue. This growth, along with other adaptations, enables your muscles to exert more force.

MUSCULAR ENDURANCE

In contrast, your muscles adapt to *muscular endurance* training by improving your aerobic enzymes and developing more capillaries and larger and more numerous mitochondria. These adaptations improve your body's delivery and use of oxygen within muscle fiber. Thus, when you do numerous repetitions, you stimulate your muscle fiber to get better at using oxygen and aerobic enzymes in order to produce energy, which in turn improves your endurance and your ability to use fat as a source of energy.

In summary, as you plan your muscular fitness program, remember that you must do different types of training in order to produce both muscular endurance and muscular strength. In addition, take care to ensure that your program is specific and relevant to your interests and activities so that your training will be meaningful.

➤ To improve your performance in cycling or skiing, develop your leg strength.

➤ To improve your running or extend your stamina in swimming, cycling, or hiking, develop your muscular endurance.

FitFact

Your training should be tailored to your goal: Do you want to gain strength, muscular endurance, or both?

You will learn how to develop a personalized muscular fitness program in chapters 6 and 7.

The table below shows that high-resistance training helps you build strength, whereas low-resistance repetitions help you develop muscular endurance. Use the table to help plan your training program. As you gain experience, you will need to increase weight to build strength, or increase weight or repetitions to build muscular endurance.

Strength Versus Muscular Endurance Training

	Strength	Muscular endurance
To develop	More force	More endurance
Prescription	8–12RM*	15–25RM
	1–3 sets**	1–3 sets
	3 days/week	3 days/week

*RM = repetition maximum, the most repetitions you can do with the weight. When you can do more than 12 (for strength) or 25 (for muscular endurance) repetitions, it is time to increase the resistance (load).

**Set = one group of 8–12 or 15–25RM; after 4 weeks do 2 sets, and after 8 weeks do 3 sets.

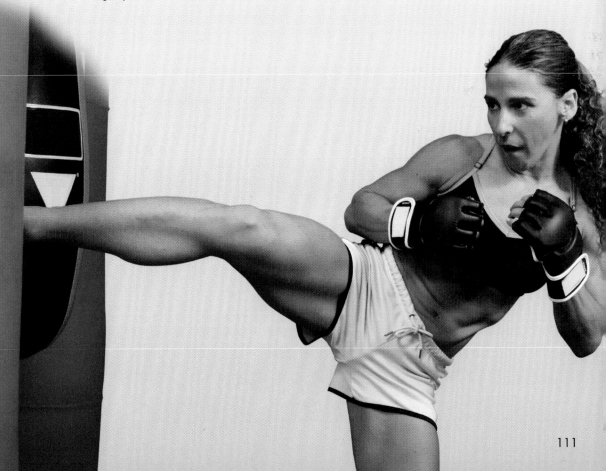

Flexibility

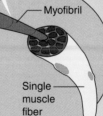

Flexibility

Flexibility is the range of motion through which your limbs can move. Your range is restricted by your skin, your connective tissue, and conditions within your joints; it can also be limited by excessive body fat. If you force a limb to move beyond its normal range, you may suffer an injury. Thus, if you improve your flexibility, you may reduce your injury risk. In addition, stretching helps you maintain range of motion that might be reduced by strength or endurance training. In fact, runners stretch to keep the activity enjoyable, since their calf, hamstring, groin, and back muscles can tighten and become sore, especially when they increase the intensity or duration of their training.

Stretching begins with the sarcomeres inside the muscle fibers. As a sarcomere stretches, the area of overlap between the thick and thin myofilaments decreases, allowing the muscle fiber to get longer. The muscle fiber is pulled out to its full length sarcomere by sarcomere. The more fibers that are stretched, the greater the length developed by the stretched muscle.

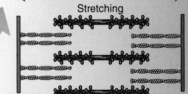

Sarcomere

Resting state

Stretching

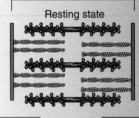

Myofibril

Single muscle fiber

In short, daily stretching can make the difference between enjoyment and discomfort, and I have found that the need for stretching increases with age. Since your range of motion is greatest when your joints and muscles are warm, it is best to do your stretching exercises after warming up—but before you engage in vigorous effort. Doing so can reduce uncomfortable feelings of tightness from previous exertion. If you also stretch *after* you exercise, during your cool-down period, you may minimize muscle soreness and enjoy greater flexibility during your next workout.

The practice of yoga has gained popularity in recent years as a safe, enjoyable way to improve flexibility and achieve relaxation or even a meditative state. When yoga is considered apart from its mystical elements, however, the benefits appear to be limited to flexibility and balance; there is little evidence to support claims that yoga improves aerobic fitness, and although it can improve muscular strength and endurance, the gains do not appear to be significant.

Many people believe that flexibility contributes to success in work and sport, and there is some truth to this view. In the workplace, lack of flexibility may be implicated in acute and chronic injuries and repetitive trauma, and it is certainly important in athletic activities that require a large range of motion (e.g., gymnastics, figure skating, or diving). Stretching can be valuable in these settings. Even so, the relationship between stretching and injury prevention is somewhat complicated. When the activity at hand consists of low-intensity movements—as in jogging, cycling, or swimming—there is less need for an extensive stretching program. Older folks may profit from regular stretching exercises, since connective tissue becomes less elastic with age.

In chapters 6 and 7, I recommend some static and dynamic flexibility exercises. I also encourage you to add more if you feel sore, if you experience tightness in your muscles or joints, or if your activity (e.g., golf, tennis, or swimming) requires a large range of motion.

Other Components of Muscular Fitness

Now that you've learned about strength, muscular endurance, and flexibility, consider whether you want to add any of the following additional components of muscular fitness to your program: speed, power, balance, agility, and neuromuscular coordination. These elements—particularly agility and balance—are often important in sport and in work, and they may help you reduce your risk of serious injury.

Speed and Power

Speed and power are important and related components of sport. Both involve muscular strength, and both can be improved. Speed—possibly the most exciting element in sport—requires the contraction of fast-twitch muscle fibers to provide rapid acceleration. Power, in turn, is a combination of speed and strength (force). We can define power as work divided by time, or the rate of doing work. Thus, a person who is able to do more work than someone else in the same unit of time has more power.

Power is essential to success in a number of sports. Some of them are obvious, such as football, in which a lineman must use explosive power in order to move his opponent out of the way. But power is also important in any sport that calls for speed and acceleration—even cycling and cross-country skiing. Lance Armstrong, for example, wins races because he generates more power than his competitors do in sprints and uphill climbs.

Though prominent in sport, power is seldom required of nonathletic adults. If you decide to increase your power for use in a certain activity—whether it be cycling, skiing, basketball, or another sport—remember the principle of specificity. If you are a runner, for instance, you can increase your running power by lifting weights, running uphill, or running against resistance. (You can increase your speed through high-speed repetitions or running downhill.) For more about power, consult the bibliography, especially Sharkey and Gaskill (2006).

Balance

Balance can be static or dynamic. Static balance is your ability to keep your balance while you are not moving. It can be measured by doing the stork stand, in which you stand on one foot with your hands on your hips and your eyes closed. Young adults typically exceed 40 seconds in this position, whereas elderly persons average a few seconds at best. Static balance is important in various activities, including mountain climbing, maintaining balance on a steep mountain bike climb, and keeping your balance on a ladder. Though it declines with age—as well as inactivity, illness, or head injury—you can improve your balance through specific training. In addition, because the decline in static balance with age increases your risk of falls, it is important for older persons to maintain a well-lit house and use a nightlight to make late-night movements safer.

Dynamic balance, on the other hand, is your ability to maintain equilibrium while you are in motion. In other words, it's your ability to stay balanced even as you move around your office or kitchen, walk up and down stairs, or play a sport. Surprisingly, some of us have poor static balance but fairly good dynamic balance.

balance

All balance depends on your ability to integrate visual input with information derived from balance receptors in your inner ear and from receptors in your muscles and joints. Static and dynamic balance both contribute to performance in sport and in life.

You can improve your balance by participating in sports and other movement activities (e.g., tai chi or yoga). Leg strength is a factor in dynamic balance, especially in older persons, and research has found that elderly tai chi practitioners exhibited better balance than sedentary subjects. Their balance was about the same, however, as that found in a group of elderly golfers, and a separate study found that active senior males who participated in a balance intervention program showed little improvement in static or dynamic balance. It would appear, then, that simply leading an active life may help maintain balance, even in senior citizens.

You may recall from chapter 2 that training is specific, and we think the same is true for balance. Thus, when football players take part in ballet classes, they will become better dancers, but whether they will improve their performance on the field has yet to be demonstrated. If you want to improve your balance in a specific activity (e.g., skiing), the best way to do so is to practice that activity.

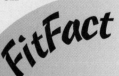

FitFact

You can improve your dynamic balance by engaging in a wide range of activities. Try tai chi or balance training to improve static balance.

Agility

Agility is the ability to change your position and direction rapidly and precisely without losing your balance. It depends on strength, speed, balance, and coordination. As you might imagine, agility is crucial in sport, and it can also help you avoid embarrassment and injury in recreational activities and in potentially dangerous work situations (e.g., construction). No single test can predict agility for all situations—it is associated with specific skills—but you can improve it with practice and experience in your chosen activity. Neither extreme strength nor aerobic fitness improves your agility, but, for obvious reasons, excess weight hinders it. Because agility also deteriorates with fatigue, aerobic and muscular *endurance* should help you maintain agility for extended periods. They could also help older persons avoid falls and injuries.

Ruth

As you evaluate what types of activities you will do to improve your muscular fitness, you will have many choices, from traditional strength training to alternative approaches such as yoga and tai chi. Consider Ruth, a 40-year-old living on Cape Cod, who had a health problem that defied diagnosis. After she suffered many months of debilitating illness, doctors finally confirmed a case of Lyme disease, an illness transmitted by ticks common in New England forests. Treatment enabled her to recover partially, but she remained weak and unable to enjoy life. To recover further, she turned to yoga for meditative stretching and then to Pilates, a resistance and flexibility regimen that strengthens core muscles. Her progress was so slow that she sought other sources for relief, including the Feldenkrais method, a program said to improve efficiency of movement. She also practiced tai chi, a slow, flowing Chinese discipline said to improve balance, and engaged in nutritional therapy, mind–body healing, acupuncture, and physical manipulation. In time, with help from her family and friends, she became strong enough to return to near-normal status.

Ruth relied on a series of alternative therapies—techniques still undergoing scientific evaluation of their effectiveness. She also could have used the services of a physical therapist, an exercise physiologist, a certified fitness instructor, or a local health club. Remember that exercise is exercise—for example, you can improve lower-body flexibility through traditional static stretching, tai chi, or any number of other recreational activities. Use alternative therapies if you wish to and can afford them, but remember that your body responds to the exercise, not to the cost of a given program.

Coordination or Skill

Coordination involves a smooth flow of movement as you execute a task. In hitting a tennis serve, for example, you generate force through a sequence of movements. You develop momentum from turning your body, then, as that momentum peaks, extend your arm at the elbow, and finally deliver maximum racquet speed with a snap of your wrist. However, if the forces are applied in the wrong sequence, your movement is uncoordinated and fails to deliver the desired result.

Though a certain amount of coordination may be inherited, skill is generally achieved through practice, practice, and more practice. If you repeatedly perform the *wrong* movement, however, you will develop bad habits that are hard to break. Thus, practice is not merely a matter of effort. It is crucial to ensure that you are practicing properly. If you are uncertain of proper technique, seek professional instruction.

Because every skill is specific, each one must be learned individually. Being good at tennis doesn't guarantee that you will be good at badminton, squash, or racquetball; sure, they all involve a racket, but we now know that skill does not transfer between sports as readily as we once thought. As you train for fitness, you will discover another feature of coordination or skill: Skilled individuals don't waste movement or energy; they work efficiently. A skilled runner uses less energy than an unskilled runner moving at the same speed. Similarly, a skilled worker often outproduces a stronger but less skilled co-worker. This is good news! Skill, coordination, and technique can be learned, and you can use them to make good use of leverage and of your large muscle groups, thereby minimizing fatigue and injury of your smaller muscles.

Keys to Muscular Fitness

➤ Improve your muscular fitness to improve your health and performance.

➤ Training is specific: Know what you are training for in order to maximize your gains in muscular fitness.

➤ Improve your strength and muscular endurance to enhance your enjoyment of meaningful activities.

➤ Muscular fitness can enhance your balance, coordination, and performance.

What's Next?...

Now that you know more about muscular fitness, move on to chapter 6 to discover how to improve your strength and muscular endurance.

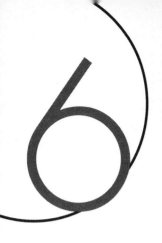

6

Muscular Fitness Training

Shape Yourself

You must be true to yourself. Strong enough to be true to yourself. Brave enough to be strong enough to be true to yourself. Wise enough to be brave enough to be strong enough to shape yourself from what you actually are.

~ Sylvia Constance Ashton-Warner

Mary

had gone through a tough time,

first in dealing with her rebellious teenage daughter, and then in supporting her husband as he confronted the loss of his job. She developed mild depression, and in the process gained weight and lost muscle tone. Over time, as she learned how to handle her daughter and got used to the new part-time job she took on to help support the family, Mary vowed to regain a healthy, active body. She increased her physical activity and limited her caloric intake in order to lose weight.

Mary

...regain a healthy, active body

She returned to the health club and resumed muscular fitness training to regain muscle tone. And she targeted specific muscles to improve her posture and appearance. In short, Mary undertook the process of reshaping her body. Before long, she regained her trim figure, and she and her husband were walking, cycling, dancing, and loving life together.

5 LB

SHAPING

Like Mary in our opening story, you can take steps to shape your body. These techniques will not allow you to overcome genetic characteristics or the inevitable effects of aging, but they will enable you to improve your posture and appearance—and look better in clothing or a bathing suit.

Here are the steps to follow:

1. Lose excess weight.
2. Improve muscle tone.
3. Improve posture.
4. Increase muscle size.

Lose excess weight. Weight loss requires you to burn more calories than you consume. To burn calories, increase your aerobic activity (e.g., through walking or cycling); at the same time, eat less—in particular, less of high-calorie desserts, dressings, and snacks. As your fitness improves, you will be better able to burn calories. See chapter 8 for more on losing fat and controlling your body weight.

Improve muscle tone. When muscle is used, it becomes taut and firm, so you should engage in a variety of activities and in concerted muscular fitness training to tone your muscles. Be sure to incorporate core training and stretching into your program.

tone

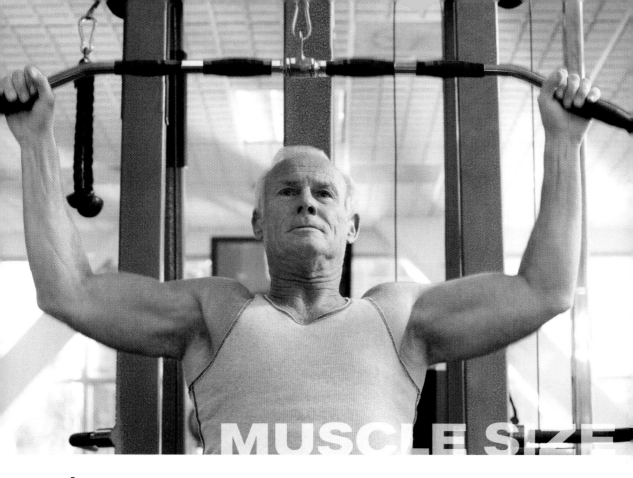

MUSCLE SIZE

Improve posture. As you lose weight and improve muscle tone, begin to pay attention to your posture. When you stand erect with your head up and shoulders back, you look and feel better. Core training improves your posture, and rowing exercises help pull your shoulders back.

Increase muscle size. Strength training can increase the size of your skeletal muscles. You will enjoy the best results if you do several sets of 10 to 15 repetition maximum, that is, use the heaviest weight that you can lift 10 to 15 times. Speaking generally, men often like to increase the size of their biceps, triceps, pectoral (chest), and abdominal muscles. Women may focus in particular on pectoral and abdominal exercises to improve their appearance in a dress or bathing suit, though, like men, they may also enjoy having strong, attractive arms!

This shaping program will certainly improve your appearance. Just remember that it may take many months of weight loss and training to bring about major changes in appearance. As you make progress toward your goals, your success will reinforce your efforts.

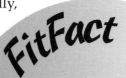

Hypertrophy is an increase in muscle mass (cross-sectional area, or size, of muscle) due to an increase in the size of individual muscle fibers.

Evaluating Your Muscular Fitness

Muscular fitness contributes to health and performance. It makes you better able, for example, to do yardwork, hike with a backpack, cycle or run uphill, paddle a canoe, or ski. What's more, the benefits grow with time. See what muscular fitness can do for you!

You may prefer to do some training before doing a fitness test, but if you're wondering just how your muscular fitness measures up right now, you can find out by doing any of a number of established tests. I've included some in the table below. The best tests are ones that mimic the movements common to the activity for which you are training. If you decide to do a vigorous test, remember to warm up and do some stretching beforehand.

Muscular Fitness Tests

Fitness component	Test used	MEN			WOMEN		
		Low	Medium	High	Low	Medium	High
Strength (upper body)	Chin-up*	<6	6–10	>10	<20	20–30	>30
Muscular endurance (upper body)	Push-up	<20	20–40	>40	<10	10–20	>20
Muscular endurance (trunk)	Sit-up	<30	30–50	>50	<25	25–40	>40
Strength (legs)	Leg press**	<220%	220–320%	>320%	<220%	220–300%	>300%
Flexibility	Sit and reach: Can you reach your toes?	No	Yes	Beyond	No	Yes	Beyond
Power	Vertical jump***	<17 inches	17–23 inches	>23 inches	<10 inches	10–15 inches	>15 inches
Speed (40 meters)	40-meter sprint (measured in seconds)	>7.5	7.5–6.0	<6.0	>9.0	9.0–7.5	<7.5

*Women do modified chin-up (bar is chest high; heels remain on ground).

**Percent of body weight.

***Low vertical jump is associated with a low percentage of fast-twitch fibers.

Adapted by permission from Sharkey and Gaskill, 2007, p. 149.

How did you do? In what areas would you like to improve? Consider your training goals and the results of the tests as you begin to develop a muscular fitness training program.

What Are Your Muscular Fitness Goals?

What is the best way to train for strength or muscular endurance? The answer depends on what you are training to accomplish—that is, on your training goal. Let's take some time now to figure out your goal: Is it strength or endurance? Check all the boxes on page 130 that apply to you.

My Muscular Fitness Goals

Muscular Strength

- ❏ I would like to be able to lift heavy loads (e.g., children, heavy bags of groceries, or suitcases) without risk of injury.
- ❏ I'd like to strengthen my arms in order to improve my swimming or my tennis game.
- ❏ I'd like to improve my sport performance (e.g., generate more power when I swing a softball bat or hit a golf ball or volleyball).
- ❏ I want to be able to climb steep hills on my bicycle.
- ❏ I'd like to be better able to pull, push, lift, and carry—whether it's carrying groceries, pushing dirt in a wheelbarrow, or pulling a suitcase through an airport.
- ❏ I want to have the strength in my fingers, hands, and forearms to open cans, jars, and bottles on my own.

Muscular Endurance

- ❏ I want to be able to lift objects (e.g., children, groceries, or boxes) repeatedly without tiring.
- ❏ I would like to be able to carry heavy objects for longer periods of time or for greater distances than I currently can.
- ❏ I'd like to be able to run longer and faster.
- ❏ I'd like my legs to hold up for long-distance hikes or bike rides, or even just when standing a long time.
- ❏ I'd like to have more energy to run and play with my kids.
- ❏ I want to do household tasks such as painting walls, working in the yard, changing light bulbs or smoke alarms, and moving lightweight furniture without fatiguing.
- ❏ I'd like to be able to go up and down flights of stairs without getting winded.
- ❏ I'd like to have arm and leg stamina that lasts for an entire basketball game or volleyball or tennis match.
- ❏ I'd like to increase the stamina in my arm, wrist, and finger muscles in order to improve my ability to play a musical instrument.

As you evaluate the items you marked, does one set of goals seem more urgent or impactful to you, or are they about the same? This will give you an idea of whether you might want to train for strength, muscular endurance, or both.

Which Muscles Should You Train?

Now that you know whether you want to train for strength or muscular endurance or a little of both, you need to think about which muscles to train. Consider your training goals, and then determine which muscles are the prime movers—the most important for the specific skill or task. Next, determine which muscles offer assistance, and which are needed to maintain muscle balance (e.g., balance of strength in quadriceps and hamstring muscles). Notice from the table on page 132 that the assisting muscles and muscles needed for muscle balance are sometimes different and sometimes the same. If conducting this analysis seems too difficult, consult a coach, trainer, or fitness instructor. Remember that you must also identify essential stretching and core training (trunk) exercises to support your progress.

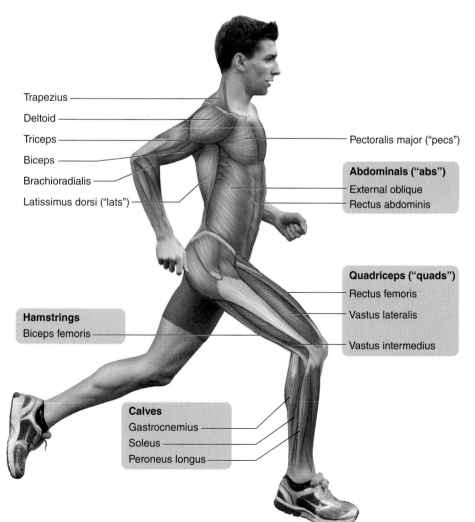

Trapezius

Deltoid

Triceps

Biceps

Brachioradialis

Latissimus dorsi ("lats")

Pectoralis major ("pecs")

Abdominals ("abs")
External oblique
Rectus abdominis

Quadriceps ("quads")
Rectus femoris
Vastus lateralis
Vastus intermedius

Hamstrings
Biceps femoris

Calves
Gastrocnemius
Soleus
Peroneus longus

131

For example, to improve hiking strength and endurance, you might identify these muscles and exercises:

Sample Analysis for Improving Strength and Muscular Endurance for Hiking

Body part	Muscle function	Exercise	Improvement
Legs	Prime movers: quadriceps (front of thighs)	Leg press	Strength
		Hiking with a pack, mountain biking	Endurance
	Assisting muscles: gluteals	Leg press, squat	Strength
	Muscle balance: hamstrings (back of thighs)	Leg flexion	Strength
Upper body	Prime movers: triceps	Dip, push-up, triceps extension	Muscular endurance with hiking poles
	Assisting muscles: biceps	Curl, chin-up	Strength to lift a pack

What Is Overload?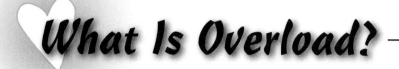

The overload principle in muscular fitness training states the following:

- In order to improve, you must overload a body system—that is, impose a demand on it. For instance, to increase strength, you have to impose a demand that exceeds two-thirds of a muscle's maximal force.
- As your body adapts to loading, you have to increase the load if you want to continue improving.
- Improvements depend on the intensity (tension for strength), duration (repetitions), and frequency of your training.

FitFact

Use a spotter when lifting heavy free weights.

The bench press overloads the pectoral and triceps muscles.

How to Train

If you just want to get stronger or gain muscular endurance for health reasons or to remain independent, almost any method will work. There is no best method for strength or muscular endurance training. Here are some options, depending on your level of experience:

➤ **Beginner.** If you're new to muscular fitness training, you will make progress easily. Start by using resistance bands or light weights. Don't fall into the trap of purchasing the latest equipment advertised in infomercials. Instead, try some traditional and inexpensive equipment (e.g., using hand weights at home or visiting a fitness club) to see what suits your interests. Then branch out from there.

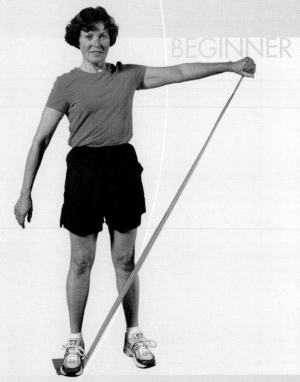

BEGINNER

◄ **Intermediate.** Intermediates need more resistance in order to make progress, so if you fall into this category, you'll do well with calisthenics and weight machines, which are convenient and require less supervision than free weights do.

INTERMEDIATE

➤ **Advanced.** If you have trained with weights for a long time, you probably already know that your best bets are weight machines and free weights. Though free weights are inexpensive and versatile, they require you to have a spotter or some kind of supervision for safety. For many muscle groups, you can get good results from weight machines.

ADVANCED

Begin with simple equipment and move to machines and free weights as you make progress. As you gain experience, you may want to purchase resistance equipment for home use.

If you want to gain strength to improve your performance at work or in playing a sport, your training should be *specific* to your goal. We conducted a study at the University of Montana in which college women trained with either weights or calisthenics. The weight group did best on lifting tests, and the calisthenics group scored best on calisthenics tests. This study showed how important it is to train in the manner in which you plan to use the strength you develop. If you want to increase the distance of your drive in golf, do resistance training with the muscles used in the swing. In addition, be sure you do core training (see page 145) to strengthen your trunk and reduce your risk of injury.

Be sure the training program you adopt is appropriate for your level of fitness and ability. What is best for beginners doesn't work for athletes, and vice versa. I address this further in chapter 7.

FitFact

Make sure your muscular fitness training program matches your fitness level and abilities and trains the muscles you want to train.

Muscle Soreness

If you overdo training, you may experience soreness 24 hours later. According to current thinking, this delayed-onset muscle soreness (DOMS) has several possible causes: slight tears in connective tissue, damage to muscle fiber, accumulation of fluid (edema), uncontrolled contractions of muscle fibers, or lingering effects of metabolic by-products—though not, contrary to what many think, lactic acid, which is eliminated within an hour after your workout. And we know that exercise involving eccentric contraction—as in downhill running or lowering a heavy weight—is more likely to cause soreness that persists for days and reduces your enjoyment of subsequent activity.

You can minimize soreness by practicing patience. Avoid maximal lifting; instead, begin with light weights and progress gradually. Also steer clear of all-out running and ballistic movements such as hard throwing when you begin or renew an activity. At the same time, since experience shows that we are seldom patient enough, we also need a way to reduce soreness, and stretching has been shown to reduce muscle discomfort. It is worth your while to stretch before and after exercise, or anytime that you feel tight or sore.

If your muscles are sore, you may experience reduced strength for as long as 2 weeks. You'll find that you recover faster and have less soreness after successive bouts of exercise. Fortunately, DOMS occurs only during the start-up phase, and the symptoms disappear within a few weeks, reappearing only after a long layoff or the vigorous start of a new activity. Indeed, exercise-induced muscle soreness seems to inoculate the body against subsequent discomfort for up to 6 months following the initial soreness.

In overtrained muscle, microscopic tears in the muscle membrane allow the leakage of creatine kinase.

Stiffness

Swelling

Pain

Loss of strength

Improving Strength and Muscular Endurance

Strength does not increase rapidly, but if you stick with a good program, you will be gratified with the results. Generally, you can expect to increase your strength by 1 to 3 percent per week. If you've never trained for strength, you will progress faster. If you combine strength training with strenuous aerobic training, you will progress slower. In any case, your rate of improvement will plateau as you approach your potential maximal strength. Remember that you will gain strength only in the muscle groups you train. You should also pay attention to your diet. Your progress will be slowed if you fail to consume adequate protein and energy (calories). If you are following a weight-loss diet, be sure to consume sufficient protein. If you have been sedentary up until now, and if you eat an adequate diet, you can reasonably expect to increase your strength by 50 percent or more in 6 months!

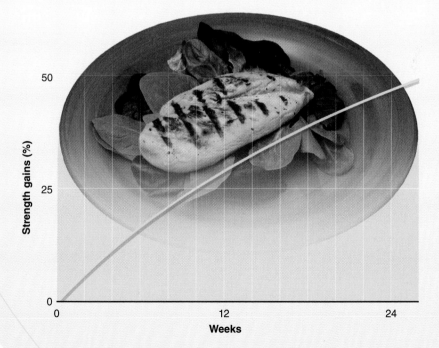

With strength training, your strength gains will be high at first and then will level off as you near your maximal strength. Keep at it! You can increase your strength by 50 percent or more in 6 months.

Muscular endurance is highly trainable. When you have enough strength to do a given task, you can improve your muscular endurance with relative ease. It is difficult, for example, to progress from 2 to 4 chin-ups (which takes strength) but easy to improve from 20 to 40 push-ups (which takes muscular endurance). In one study in our lab at the University of Montana, participants improved their muscular endurance by 10 percent per week when they trained with 15 to 25 repetition maximum. In addition, on an upper-body endurance test, subjects who performed muscular endurance training improved their muscular endurance by 70 percent versus just 50 percent for those who did strength training. The benefits of improving muscular endurance are considerable. Assuming you have adequate strength, your enjoyment of and performance in most activities will be enhanced if you improve your muscular endurance. Consider, for example, tennis and skiing. If you want to do well at either, you will need to invest hours of practice, which in turn requires muscular endurance. If you are tired, you are likely to practice poorly on the tennis court or face increased injury risk on the slopes.

Maintaining Strength and Muscular Endurance

If you keep your training intensity (resistance) high, you can maintain your strength even at a lower volume and frequency of training. Specifically, you can maintain strength for 6 weeks or more by performing one session per week, and you can maintain it for an extended period if you do two sessions per week. Muscular endurance, on the other hand, is easily maintained with one session per week. As you get older, you will want to engage in a maintenance program, if only to slow the effects of aging. After age 55 or so, you will need two or more training sessions per week to slow the loss of strength and muscular endurance with age.

Flexibility

Another important aspect of muscular fitness is flexibility. Have you ever had trouble reaching high enough or far enough without experiencing muscle stress? Have you ever stretched a muscle or ligament in a way that causes pain?

If so, you might need to improve your flexibility, which in turn can improve your performance and reduce your risk of injury.

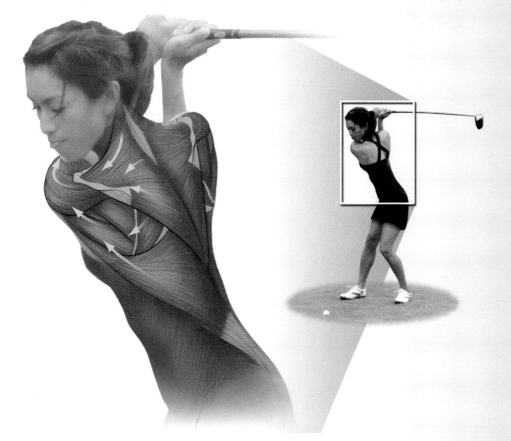

Muscles are covered with tough connective tissue, which, along with the structures of the joint and tendons, restricts how much you can move. You can greatly expand these limits through flexibility training, and doing so offers sizable benefits. As you age, or if you become inactive, your flexibility will decrease, and you will be more likely to experience injury. Low-back problems, for example, are associated with poor flexibility of the back and hamstrings and with weak abdominal muscles. Enhanced flexibility, on the other hand, may not only reduce your injury risk but also improve your range of motion in activities such as golf, tennis, and swimming.

You should stretch after your body is warmed up.

Stretching can be static or dynamic—that is, it can involve easy movement or light bobbing. Avoid vigorous movement, which increases your risk of injury. Vigorous stretching invokes the stretch reflex, which involves a rapid stretch that causes muscle contraction rather than relaxation. That's the opposite of what you want! Instead, enjoy the gentle act of static and dynamic stretching.

When your muscles and joints are warmer,

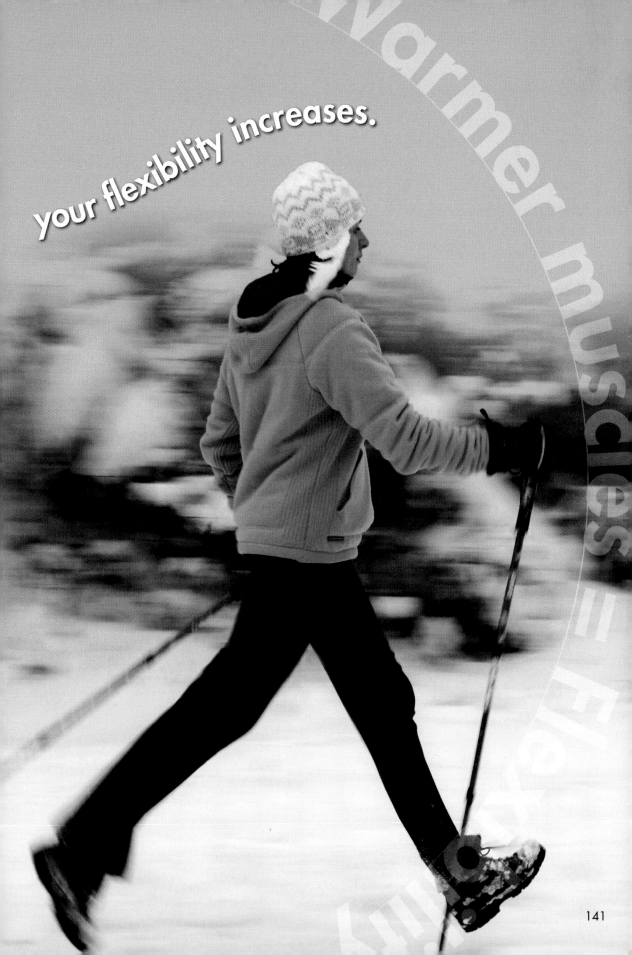

your flexibility increases.

Warmer muscles = flex...

Three Types of Stretching

1 **Static stretching** calls on you to make a slow movement to reach the point of stretch, hold the position for 5 to 10 seconds, and then relax. You may repeat the stretch up to 3 times and bob very lightly.

2 **Contract-and-relax stretching** is a variation of static stretching. Here, you perform a static stretch, relax, contract the muscle for a few seconds, and then repeat the static stretch. Contract-and-relax stretching can help you relax the muscle in order to better stretch the tendon. Using this form of stretching on your calf muscle, for example, helps reduce tightness before a run and reduces lingering muscle soreness.

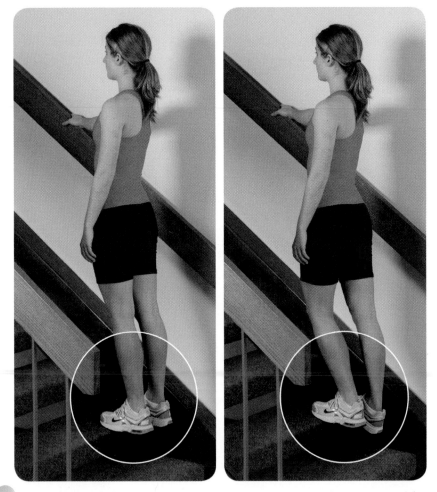

The static calf stretch (page 157) can also be done using the contract-and-relax method: Stand on the edge of a stair step with your weight on the balls of your feet; use the banister for balance. Stretch your calf by allowing one heel to sink below the edge of the step; next, contract the calf of the same leg to raise your body, and then relax back into the stretching position. Do 8 repetitions, and then switch to the other side. This is a great stretch for runners.

Dynamic stretching involves stretching in motion, often in sport-specific motions. For example, you might do arm swings that mimic the movements in golf or tennis. Thus, dynamic stretching improves your range of motion in movements directly related to performance. It may even reduce your risk of injury.

Try a dynamic stretch to prepare for your favorite activity. See chapter 7 for more examples.

Follow these how-tos for stretching:

➤ Warm up a bit with light exercise or calisthenics before you stretch.

➤ After a light warm-up, use the stretching techniques described here and in chapter 7.

➤ Finish your warm-up with more vigorous activity (*not* vigorous stretching!), or, if you prefer, begin your run or other exercise at a modest pace.

➤ Never substitute skill rehearsal, such as doing tennis strokes, for stretching.

➤ Do your warm-up and stretching before you begin to compete.

Flexibility

If you do flexibility training correctly, the results can last for a long time. In fact, after a few weeks of stretching, your improved range of motion should persist for at least 8 weeks. As you come to enjoy stretching, you may even get hooked on its subtle sensations and decide to try advanced forms such as yoga. If not, that is fine, but stay committed to doing the stretches you need to do in order to minimize soreness, reduce your injury risk, and avoid low-back problems (by stretching your back and hamstrings).

Core Training

Core training is an essential facet of muscular fitness. It focuses on the core muscles in the central portion of your body that anchor and stabilize your arms and legs during work, sport, and recreational activities. Thus, core training is a high priority in terms of both health and performance; a moderate amount of core training is also important for low-back health. Core exercises involve the abdominal, back, chest, shoulder, and hip muscles.

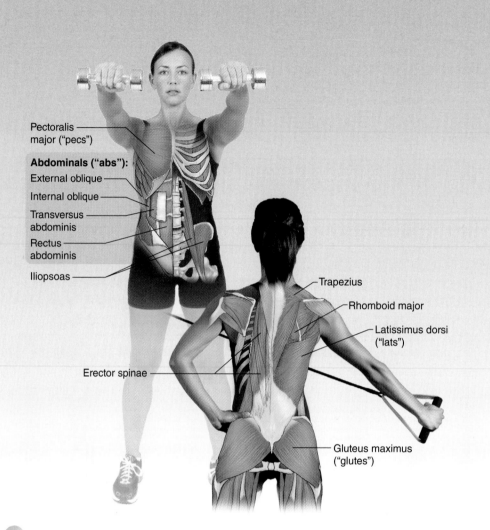

Pectoralis major ("pecs")

Abdominals ("abs"):
External oblique
Internal oblique
Transversus abdominis
Rectus abdominis
Iliopsoas

Erector spinae

Trapezius
Rhomboid major
Latissimus dorsi ("lats")

Gluteus maximus ("glutes")

The muscles of your core.

If you develop a strong core, you will enjoy a more stable trunk that is better able to transfer power from your legs and trunk to your arms, thereby reducing your risk of injury. Core stability is part of the chain of power required for you to throw, swing, lift, and perform other motions that depend on transferring power—often from your legs upward through your trunk to your arms. A well-trained core distributes the forces effectively and reduces your risk of back injury.

FitFact

Core training focuses on the central part of your body and reduces your risk of back injury.

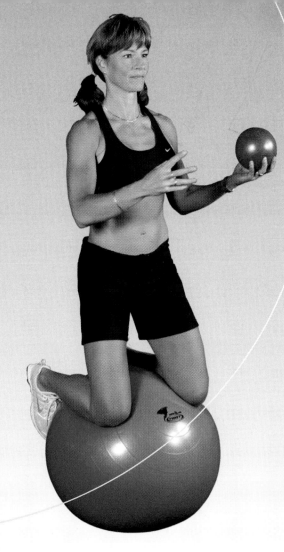

You can choose from a number of inexpensive approaches to training your core; options range from old-fashioned calisthenics and medicine balls to stability balls and Pilates. I recommend a basic program in chapter 7, which provides instructions and photos of popular core exercises. You can also use videos, books, and magazine articles to expand your use of core training.

Keys to Muscular Fitness Training

➤ Evaluate your muscular fitness.

➤ Select the muscles you will train.

➤ Decide whether these muscles need strength or muscular endurance.

➤ Select your mode of training (e.g., free weights or weight machine).

➤ Include stretching and core training in your program.

➤ Minimize muscle soreness by increasing load gradually.

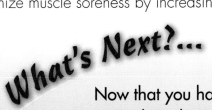

Now that you have figured out your goals for strength and muscular endurance training, move on to chapter 7 to design your personalized muscular fitness program.

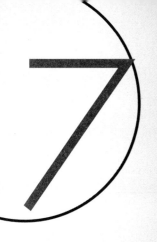

Muscular Programs

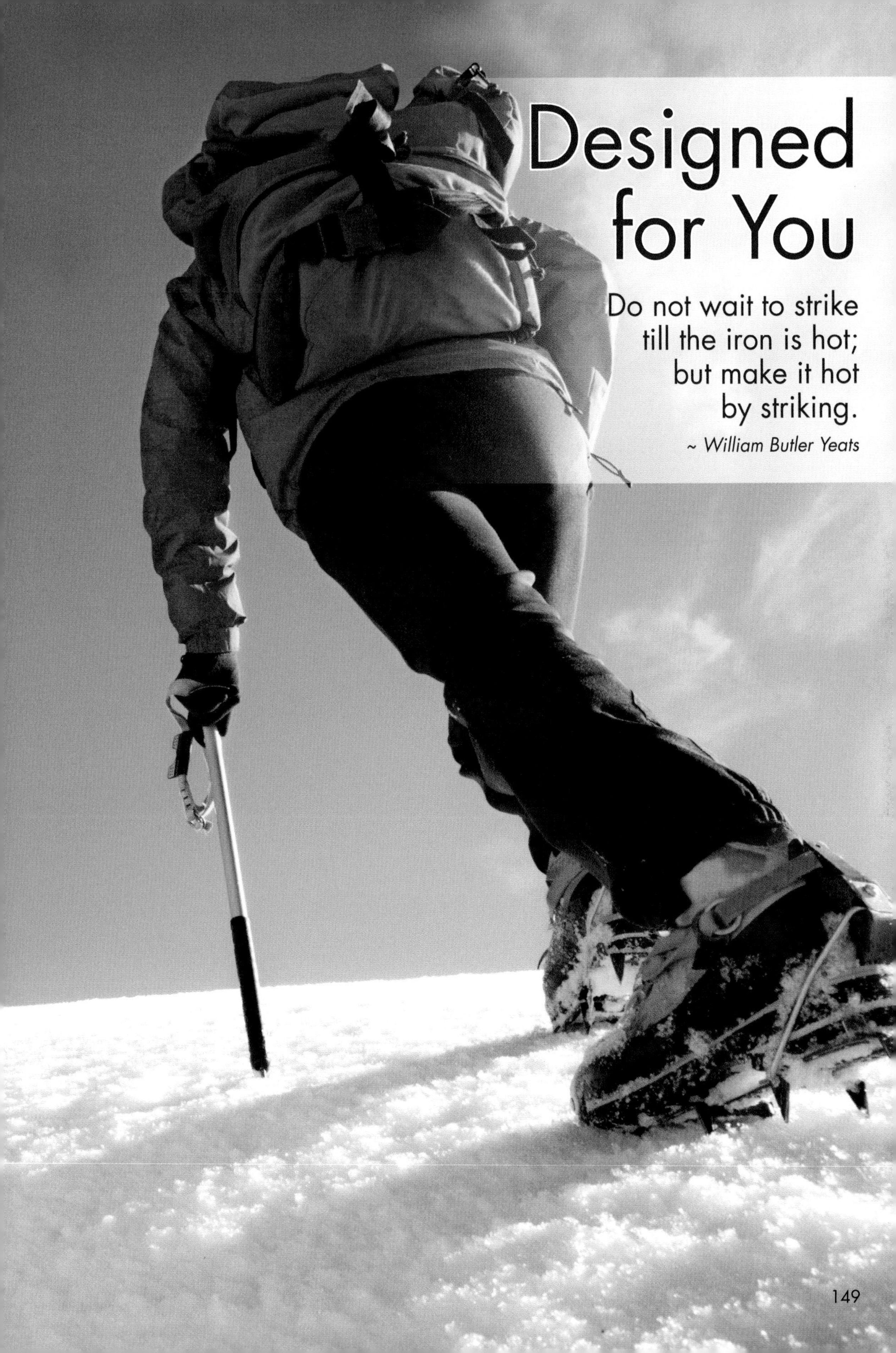

Designed for You

Do not wait to strike
till the iron is hot;
but make it hot
by striking.

~ William Butler Yeats

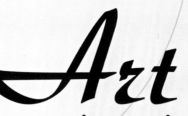

Art

is an active, muscular outdoorsman

who enjoys long backpacking, cycling, and cross-country skiing trips when he can get away from work to do them. A couple of years ago, he was injured while serving as a smoke jumper (parachuting into the wilderness to fight forest fires). From that point on, he suffered with low-back problems, which diminished his ability to live an active life.

He pursued a treatment plan that included rest, medication, and sometimes spinal manipulation by a chiropractor, along with a careful return to activity. Even so, Art saw only limited improvement until he was introduced to core training—stretching and abdominal and back exercises—as a low-back maintenance program. Now, things have changed markedly. As long as Art practices his program consistently, he is able to maintain the health and fitness of his back, and he has been able to return to the outdoor activities he enjoys so much.

Improve Your Fitness

Regardless of your age, there are many good reasons for you to improve your muscular fitness, and they boil down to two considerations: form and function. Maybe you'd like to sculpt a more attractive figure or physique or improve your posture. Or perhaps you want to get stronger or develop your muscular endurance so that you can use your strength for longer periods of time. Whatever your focus, you should evaluate your muscular fitness before you decide on a program. If you are dissatisfied with your current level of muscular fitness—or if you want to enhance performance in work or sport—then select the muscle groups you wish to improve, use the activity prescriptions in this chapter, and get going!

It is also important to realize now, even if you are still young, that as you get older, your muscular fitness will contribute crucially to your muscle mass, your mobility, and your quality of life. You should begin training long before retirement—which is to say *today*—and continue for the rest of your life. And if you are at risk for osteoporosis, make no mistake about it—this is an important concern at any age, since taking countermeasures over time can save you considerable pain and inconvenience associated with this condition. You should plan a program that includes moderate weightlifting, as well as weight-bearing aerobic activity such as walking, tennis, or jogging.

Flexibility

We all need to do some stretching, if only for low-back health. Do more to minimize soreness and injury or to improve performance and enjoyment in sport or work. Incorporate stretching before every workout, and remember to stretch only after you've warmed up your body. Begin with static stretching, and then move on to other methods. You don't need to do every stretch every time: Choose exercises that stretch the joints where you have limited motion, stretches that help with low-back health (hamstring and low-back stretches), and stretches that relate to your sport or activity. Use slow stretches to minimize soreness, and then do dynamic stretches that are sport-specific.

CAUTION   Check with your doctor before stretching if you are recovering from an injury or operation; if you have knee, shoulder, or back problems; or if your doctor has placed limits on your movement.

STATIC STRETCHES

In static stretching, you use slow movement to reach a point of stretching, hold the position for 5 to 10 seconds, and then relax. Repeat the stretch 2 or 3 times.

Neck Stretch ❯

Gently turn your head to each side as far as you comfortably can and hold.

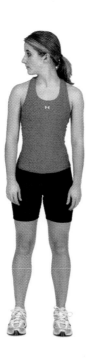

Shoulder and Arm Stretch ❯

Intertwine your fingers above your head with your palms facing upward. Push your arms upward and slightly to the rear.

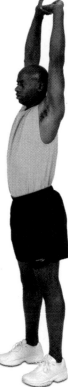

Upper-Shoulder Stretch ▶

With your right hand, grasp your left upper arm just above the elbow and pull your left arm across your chest (toward your right side).

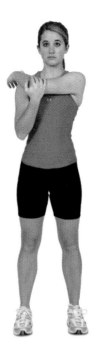

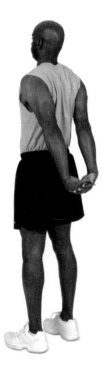

◀ Shoulder Stretch

Intertwine your fingers together behind your back. Turn your elbows inward while keeping your arms straight. Maintain an erect posture and raise your arms behind you until you feel a mild stretch.

Trunk Stretch ▶

Look over your right shoulder and turn your upper torso to the right as far as possible. Keep your hips facing forward. Repeat to the left.

VARIATION Stand 18 inches (45 cm) from a wall and face away from it. Keep your hips facing forward, rotate both hands and shoulders in one direction, and touch the wall.

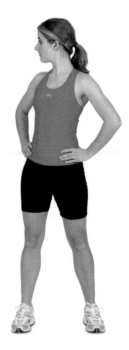

Back Stretch ❯

Hold onto a bar or other support at chest height. With your knees slightly bent, let your torso droop forward. Keep your hips directly above your feet. Try bending your knees more and experiment with holding onto objects at different heights.

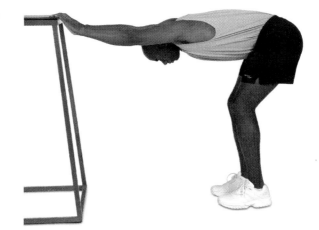

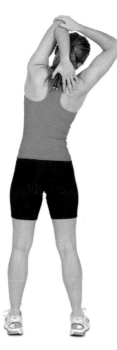

◀ Side-Bend Stretch

Stretch your left arm up and behind your head. Grasp your left elbow with your right hand and simultaneously bend to the right and pull your left arm. Repeat on the other side.

Standing Groin Stretch ❯

With your feet spread, bend your right knee while keeping your left leg straight. Do not let the knee of your bent leg go beyond your toes. Repeat on the other side.

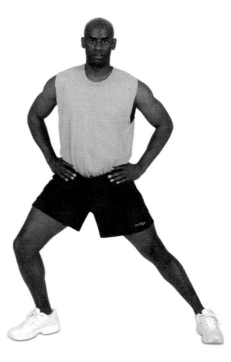

Groin and Hamstring Stretch ❯

Stand with your left side to a table or bench. Place your left heel on the bench. Gently lean toward the bench and hold that position. Repeat on the other side.

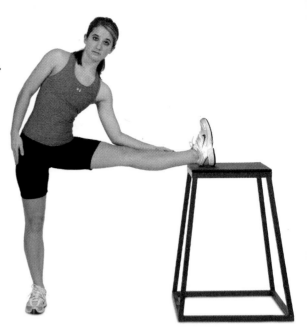

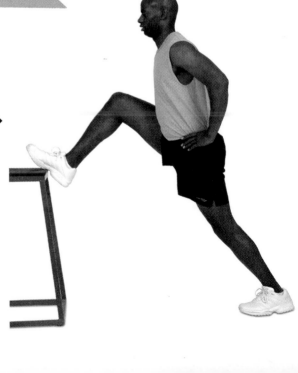

❮ Groin, Hamstring, and Hip Stretch

Place your right knee directly above your right ankle and extend your rear leg behind you. Your weight should be on the toes and ball of your rear foot. Let your torso relax forward, past your front knee. Use your hands for balance. Repeat on the other side.

Groin, Hamstring, and Front-of-Hip Stretch ❯

Place the ball of your foot on a secure, fixed surface. Keep your support leg and foot pointed forward. Push your hips toward your front foot while bending your front knee. Repeat on the opposite side.

Calf Stretch ▶

Lean against a wall or other solid support. Place most of your weight on your rear foot and push your hips down and forward while keeping your rear leg straight and your heel on the ground. Repeat on the other leg.

VARIATION   Relax your hips and push your rear knee forward and down while keeping your heel on the ground in order to stretch your lower calf.

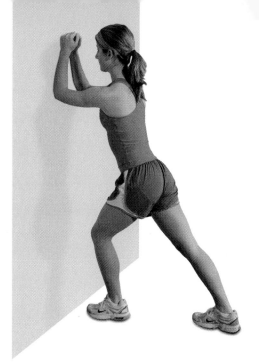

Contract-and-relax stretching. Do a static stretch (any of the stretches in this section), and then relax; next, contract the muscle for a few seconds, and then repeat the static stretch. The contract-and-relax technique helps your muscle relax so that you get a better stretch.

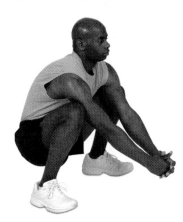

◀ Squat Stretch

Squat down with your feet flat, your knees above your toes, and your toes pointing out slightly.

VARIATION   Change the amount of spacing between your feet or between your knees.

Upper-Hamstring and Hip Stretch ▶

Hold onto the outside of your ankle (or knee, or both) and foot as shown. Gently pull your entire leg toward your torso until you feel a slight stretch in the back of your upper leg. Repeat on the other side.

VARIATION   Use your hand to gently rotate your foot through its full range of motion in order to stretch tight ligaments.

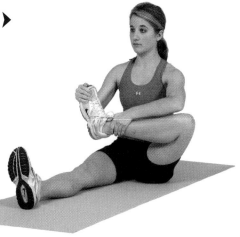

Sitting Groin Stretch ▶

Place the soles of your feet together as shown and hold onto your feet. Gently bring your torso forward by bending at your hips.

TO INCREASE THE STRETCH You can also use your elbows to gently push your knees toward the floor.

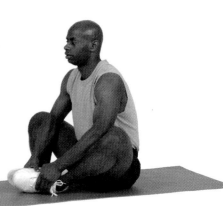

Outer-Hip Stretch ▶

Sit on the floor with one leg extended and the other bent and placed over your extended leg. Gently pull the knee of the bent leg across your torso in the direction of the opposite shoulder. Repeat on the other side.

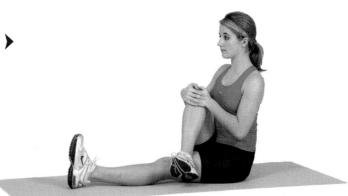

◀ Spine Stretch

Sit upright with your left leg out in front, keeping the heel flat on the floor. Bend your right leg and place your foot on the floor across your extended leg. Bend your left elbow and place it on the outside of your right thigh near your knee. Using your right arm for balance, twist while looking toward your right. Repeat on the other side.

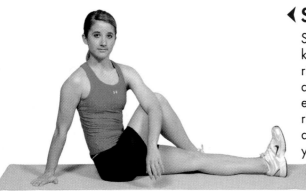

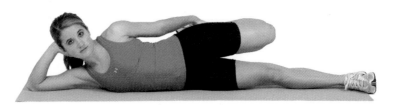

Ankle and Quad Stretch ▲

Lie on one side with your lower arm supporting your head. Hold the top of your upper foot with your free hand. Gently pull your heel toward your buttocks. Next, push the top of your foot into your hand and upward by contracting your gluteals (buttock muscles). Repeat on the other side.

DYNAMIC STRETCHES

In dynamic stretching, you move through the range of motion and work at either end of that range to increase your reach. This stretching technique mimics sports movements and uses controlled, gentle motion. Use dynamic stretching before you participate in a sport.

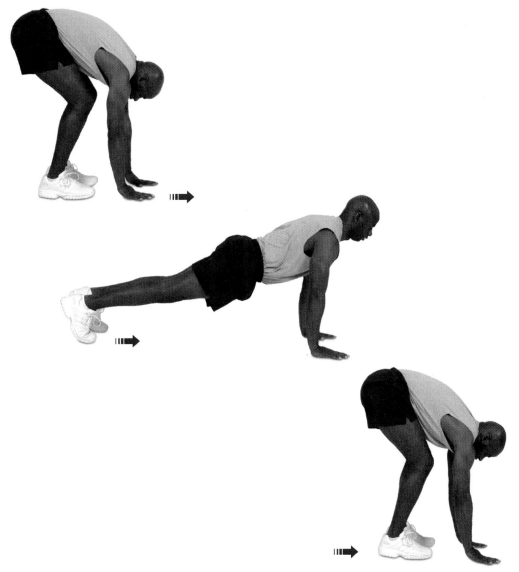

Inchworm ▲

Stand with your feet shoulder-width apart. While slightly bending your knees, bend forward at your waist and place your hands shoulder-width apart, flat on the floor. The weight of your body should be shifted back, not directly over your hands, and your buttocks should be high in the air, so that you are making an inverted V with your body. Next, move your hands alternately forward, as if taking short steps with them, until your body is in a push-up position. Then walk your legs forward to your hands, using small steps and keeping your knees slightly flexed. Repeat this motion over a distance you chose ahead of time.

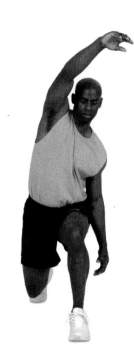

◀ Lunge With Twist

Stand with your feet parallel to each other and shoulder-width apart. Step straight forward with your left leg, bending your left knee until it is directly over your left foot. Bend your right knee slightly, lowering it until it is just above the floor. Both of your feet should be pointing straight ahead. Next, reach up with your right arm and bend your torso toward your left leg. Bring your torso back to a straight position, push off the floor by straightening the left knee, and bring your right foot up next to the left foot. After a short pause, repeat the movement starting with your right leg. Move forward with each step.

◀ Walking Knee Lift

Stand with your feet parallel to each other and shoulder-width apart. Step forward with your left leg and flex your right hip and knee to move your right thigh upward toward your chest. Grasp the front of your right knee or upper shin and use your arms to pull your right knee up farther and to squeeze your thigh against your chest. Flex your left foot upward toward your shin as your right hip and knee are flexed. Keeping your torso erect, pause for a moment, and then step down with your right leg. Shift your body weight to your right leg and repeat the motion with your left leg. Move forward with each step, increasing your range of motion and speed as you go.

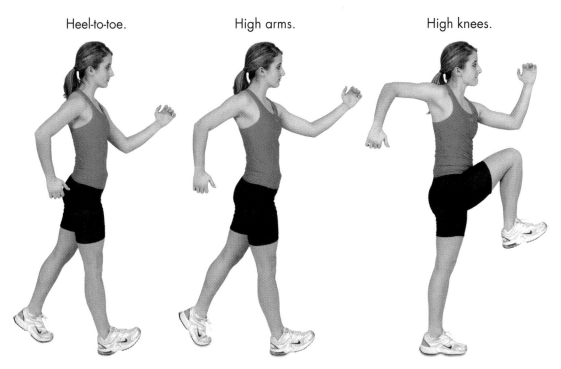

Heel-to-toe.   High arms.   High knees.

Dynamic Walking Exercises ▲

Concentrate for 6 to 8 strides (or more) on heel-to-toe walking (roll from heel to toe each time you take a step). Then transition to taking normal steps. Add an exaggerated arm swing, so that your arms swing forward and backward higher than they normally would, for 6 to 8 strides. Then switch to exaggerated knee lifts, raising each knee as high as you can, for 6 to 8 strides. Walk normally for 8 strides, and then repeat.

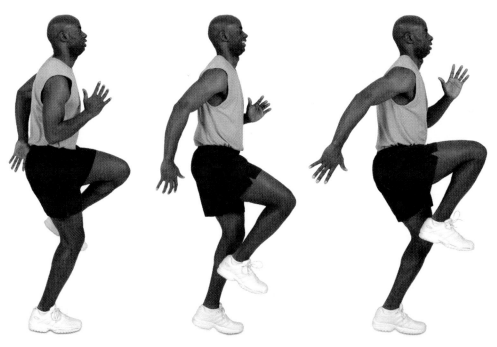

Dynamic Jogging Stretches ▲

As you jog slowly, exaggerate your knee lift and your arm swing. Try one (lift knees high), then the other (exaggerate arm swings), then both together.

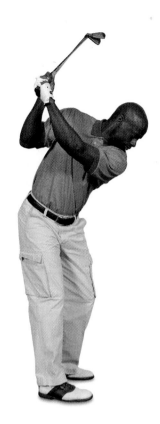

◀ Dynamic Golf Stretch

Hold two irons at their grips, assume a preparatory stance, and mimic a golf swing. Start with a low swing; then, with each swing, slowly extend the range of motion in your shoulders and hips.

Dynamic Tennis Stretch ▼

Before a match or practice session, mimic forehand and backhand swings, slowly increasing the range of motion.

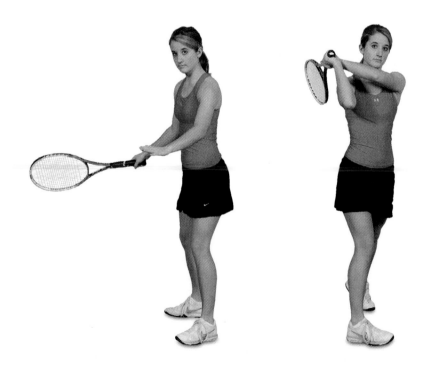

Core Training

Your core muscles—including those in your abdomen, back, hips, and shoulders—contribute to your core stability and your back health. Core training stabilizes your trunk and enhances the transfer of power to muscles in your legs and arms. For example, if you golf, improving your core stability can improve your performance and reduce your risk of injury. Core stability also minimizes fatigue in activities (e.g., tennis, cross-country skiing, or throwing) that involve transferring power through your central core.

After you do static and dynamic stretching, proceed to core training with upper and lower abdominal exercises, trunk exercises, and the rest of your core program. Change some of your core training exercises every 8 weeks as your fitness improves. Once you are satisfied with the results, develop a maintenance program. Just remember: Core training is a lifelong activity.

ABDOMINAL MUSCLES

Select one or two exercises for your abdominal muscles.

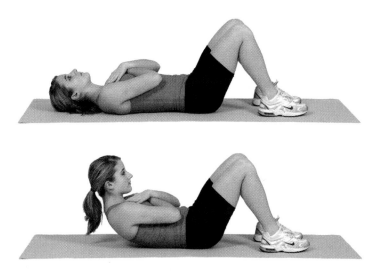

Crunch ▲

Lie on your back with your knees bent at about a 90-degree angle and your feet flat on the floor. Cross your hands over your chest and place each hand on the opposite shoulder. Do not put your hands behind your neck or head; doing so encourages neck strain. Keep your lower back flat on the floor throughout the exercise. Slowly curl your upper body, raising your head and shoulders off the floor by contracting your abdominal muscles, until your shoulder blades are 3 to 4 inches (7.5 to 10 cm) above the floor. Slowly lower your upper back until your shoulder blades touch the floor. Repeat.

Basket Hang ▶

This is an advanced abdominal exercise. Hang from the bar with an underhand grip. Raise your legs into a "basket," raising your knees as high as you can, and return to the starting position. Do as many as possible.

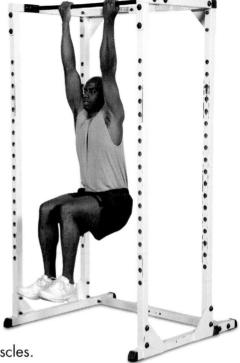

TRUNK MUSCLES

Select one or two exercises for your trunk muscles.

Leg Lift ▼

This is a good exercise for back strength and endurance. Lie facedown on the floor and, with a partner holding your trunk down, raise both legs together 5 to 10 times. Avoid hyperextension.

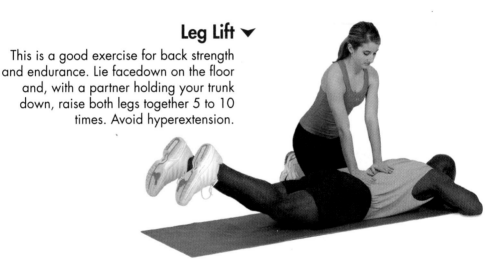

Trunk Lift ▼

Lie facedown on the floor with your fingers laced behind your head and your ankles anchored to the ground. Raise your trunk 5 to 10 times. Don't overextend.

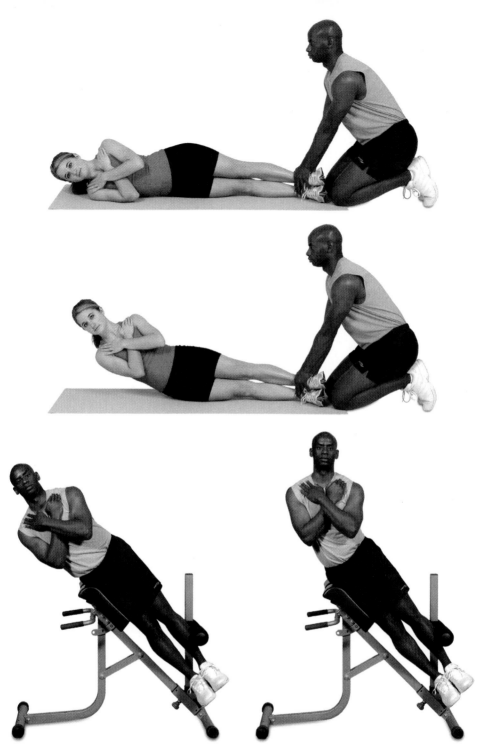

Side Trunk Lift ▲

This exercise can be done while lying either on the floor with a partner holding your ankles or on a Roman chair. Lie on your side. Have your partner hold your ankles firmly, or make sure your ankles are held securely by the machine. Cross your arms over your chest. Bending at the waist, lift your shoulders toward the ceiling. Lower your shoulders to return to the starting position. On a Roman chair, you can gradually increase the range of motion by starting from a lower position. Do 8 to 12 repetitions. Repeat on the other side. If the exercise is too easy, add a light hand weight (2.5 to 5.0 lb, or 1.1 to 2.2 kg) held in both hands at your chest or in your lower hand with your elbow bent and your upper hand on the back of your head.

HIP MUSCLES

Select one or two exercises for your hip muscles.

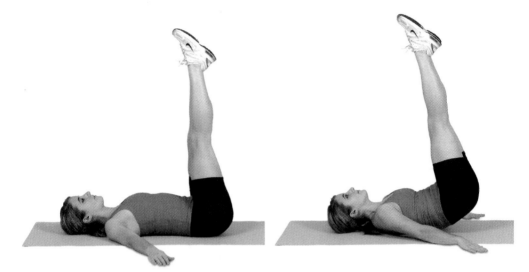

Hip Raise ▲

Lie on your back with your arms out to your sides for balance and your legs pointing straight up toward the ceiling. Raise your hips slowly. Keep your legs vertical and point your toes. Extend upward as far as possible. Slowly lower until your hips touch the ground.

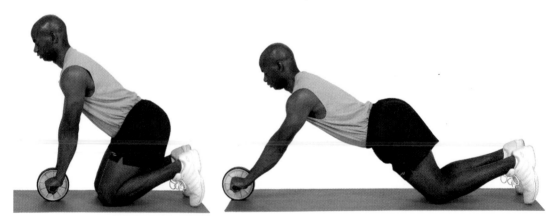

Abdominal Wheel Exercise ▲

Kneel on the edge of a mat with the abdominal wheel (a wheel with handles on each side) in front of you. Place your hands on the handles and slowly let the wheel roll forward as your body stretches out above the floor. Continue until your arms are almost fully extended or until the exercise becomes too difficult, and then return to the beginning position. Do 5 to 10 repetitions.

SHOULDER AND CHEST MUSCLES

Select one or two exercises for your shoulder and chest muscles.

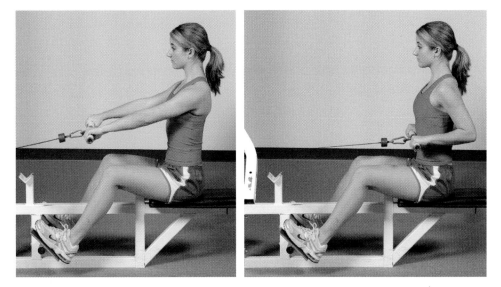

Seated Row ▲

Sit with your knees slightly flexed and hold the resistance device. Keep your upper body erect and pull the bars or bands directly toward your chest. Keep your elbows in close to your sides. Return to the starting position and repeat. Do this exercise slowly and with good control.

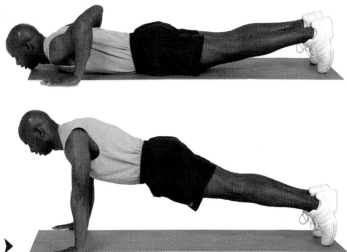

Push-Up ▶

Use push-ups as a precursor to trying the bench press. To perform a basic push-up, lie facedown on the floor with your knees fully extended and your toes pointed down to the floor. Place your hands slightly farther than shoulder-width apart with your palms down and elbows pointed outward. Keep your body in a straight line; don't allow your hips to sag or rise. Push against the floor with your hands and straighten your elbows. Lower your body by allowing your elbows to bend to a 90-degree angle. Repeat. Once you are comfortable with the conventional push-up, try doing a push-up with your feet elevated 8 to 10 inches.

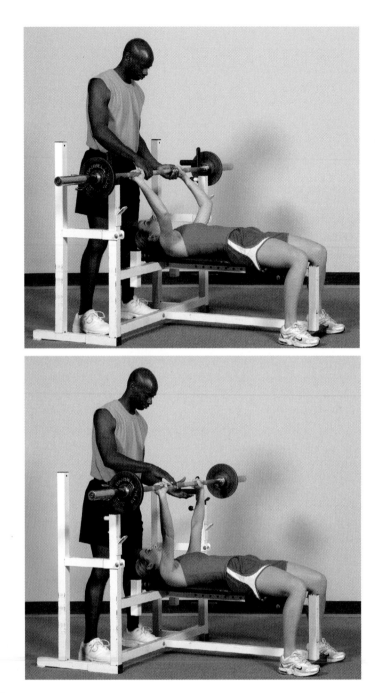

Bench Press ▲

Lie flat on your back on a bench with your feet flat on the floor. Your eyes should be directly below the racked bar. Use a closed grip (thumb wrapped around the bar) with your hands slightly farther than shoulder-width apart. Have your spotter help you move the bar off the supports. Position the bar over your chest with your elbows fully extended. Lower the bar to touch your chest. Keep your forearms perpendicular to the floor and parallel to each other. Push the bar upward until your elbows are fully extended. Do not arch your back or raise your chest. At the end of the set, ask the spotter to help you rack the bar. Keep a good grip on the bar until it is racked.

As you master this exercise, you can progress to performing it with an upward body tilt on an incline bench.

STABILITY BALL EXERCISES

Stability balls are used to add the element of balance to an exercise. Using the ball, you learn to maintain balance throughout the exercise.

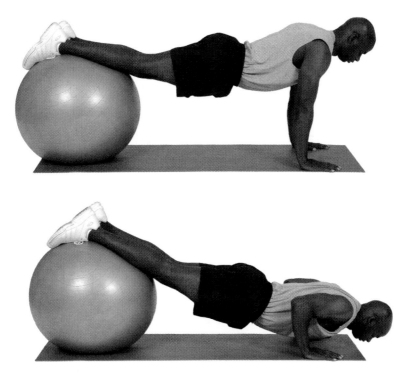

Stability Ball Push-Up ▲

Assume a push-up position with your shins and the insteps of your feet on the stability ball and your elbows fully extended. Position your feet, knees, hips, and shoulders in a straight line. Allow your elbows to flex in order to lower your face to a position that is 1 to 2 inches (2.5 to 5 cm) from the floor while keeping your body in a straight line. After reaching the lowest position, push with your arms to extend your elbows back to the starting position.

Supine Leg Curl ▶

Lie flat on your back with your arms extended out to your sides and your palms facing the floor. Lift your hips off the floor and position your lower calves and the backs of your heels on top of the stability ball. Begin the exercise with your feet, knees, hips, and shoulders in a straight line. Keeping your upper body in the same position, flex your knees (which will cause the ball to roll backward) to bring your heels toward your buttocks. Continue flexing your knees to a 90-degree angle. Keep your knees, hips, and shoulders in a straight line. After completing the leg curl, allow your knees to extend and the ball to roll forward to the starting position.

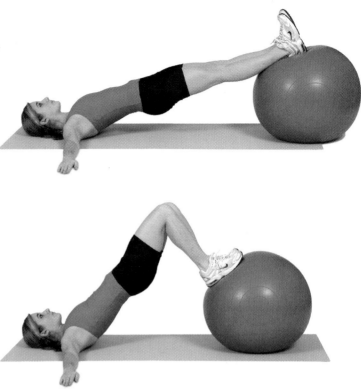

Back Hyperextension ▶

Lie facedown on the stability ball with your navel positioned on top of the ball. Place your toes on the floor at least 12 inches (30 cm) apart with your knees fully extended. Place your hands on either side of your head. Keeping your toes in contact with the floor, elevate your torso until it is fully extended (arched) and your chest is off the ball. After completing the extension, allow your torso to lower and return to the starting position.

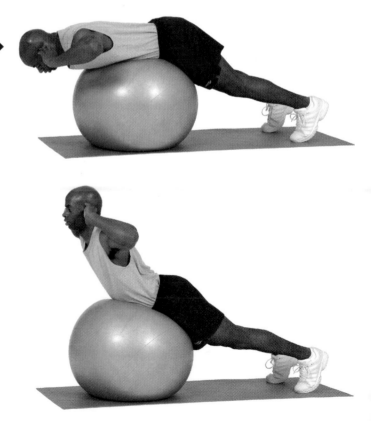

PILATES EXERCISES

Pilates is a physical fitness system developed by Joseph Pilates in Germany in the early 20th century. The program focuses on the core postural muscles that are essential to providing support for the spine.

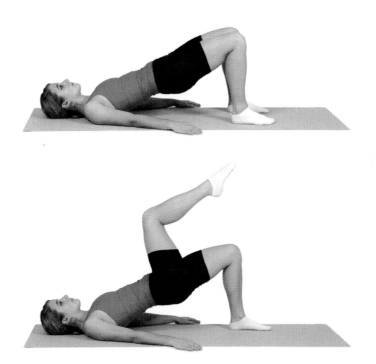

Bridge With Thigh Lift ▲

Lie on your back with your knees bent and your feet parallel to each other. Press your feet against the floor and lift your pelvis toward the ceiling to form a bridge. Exhale and lift one leg so that the thigh is about perpendicular to the floor. Inhale and lower your leg to the floor while maintaining the bridge position. Exhale and lift your other leg. Repeat.

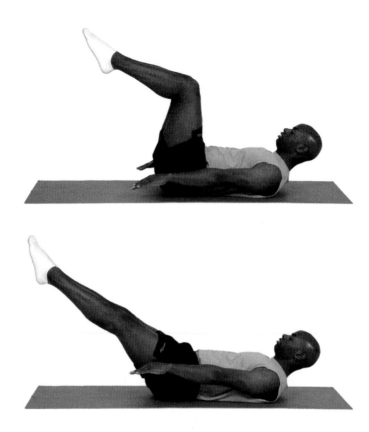

Hundred ▲

Lie on your back. Bend your knees to your chest while keeping your spine and abdominal muscles pressed toward the floor. Inhale. Exhale, then use your abdominal muscles to bring your head and your upper spine off the floor, though your shoulder blades should remain on the mat. Look toward your abdominals. Inhale. Exhale and extend your arms and legs; be sure to keep your lower back on the mat. The higher your legs, the easier the exercise. Let your legs go as low as they can without letting your body shake or moving your lower back off the mat. Keep your arms straight and low. As you take 5 short breaths in and 5 short breaths out, pump your arms up and down just a few inches in a controlled manner in unison with your breathing. If you are up to it, do 10 cycles of this, equaling 100. (One alternate method is to breathe in slowly for 5 pumps and out for 5 pumps. Another alternate method is to breathe in and out slowly while not pumping your arms at all.) Be sure to keep your shoulder blades on the mat at all times, and keep your neck and head relaxed. Let your abdominals do the work. To finish, bend your knees toward your chest, as at the beginning, to protect your back.

If you have neck or back problems, you can do this exercise with your knees bent and your feet flat on the floor. You can also do the hundred with your legs extended but with your head kept down on the floor to protect your neck. This exercise is an advanced one and not meant for an untrained individual.

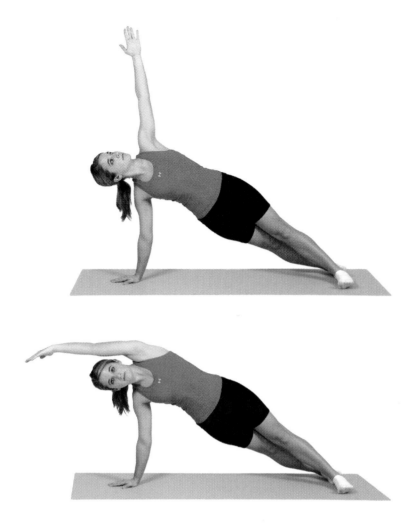

Side Bend ▲

This exercise is also more advanced than the others. Do not do this exercise if you have problems with your wrists. Sit on the floor on your right hip with your knees bent and your left leg resting on your right leg. Place your right palm on the floor while keeping your right arm straight. Support your body with your right arm; then, as you lift your left hip toward the ceiling, extend your legs so that they are straight and your left foot is resting inside your right foot. Your body should be in straight alignment from head to toe.

   Turn your head toward the ceiling. Stretch your left arm down the side of your body. Inhale and lift your left arm toward the ceiling. Then, while returning your head to the starting position (looking straight ahead), extend your left arm over (reach it over your head) so that it rests above your ear. Return your left arm to your side and lower your hips. Repeat several times, and then switch sides.

   You can make this exercise easier by putting one foot in front of the other on the mat or by leaving your bottom knee on the mat to reduce pressure on your supporting arm.

Muscular Strength and Endurance

Core training is the foundation of muscular fitness. Now it is time to move on to developing the strength and muscular endurance you need in order to accomplish the training goals you set in chapter 6. Use these guidelines to implement your program.

1 If you are new to muscular fitness training, begin with light weights, elastic bands, or calisthenics (e.g., modified push-ups).

2 After a month, you will be ready to use weight machines (where the weights are stored in a stack). Weight machines are safer than free weights and make it easy to change the resistance.

3 After some months of training, you will be ready to work with free weights. They offer more lifting options and force you to balance the load yourself. However, since free weights are not attached to a machine, your risk of injury is greater. Always use a spotter when working with free weights.

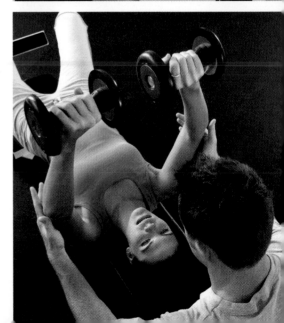

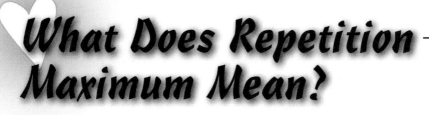

What Does Repetition Maximum Mean?

When it comes to strength training, you will find that personal trainers, Web sites, and books refer to the repetition maximum, or RM. As mentioned in chapter 5, the term 1RM refers to the maximal force you can exert in a single voluntary contraction. It's the most you can lift or pull or push one time. Because it is dangerous to attempt a true 1RM without guidance, you can begin with light weights and work your way up to the desired training level. For example, 8RM would be the heaviest weight that you can lift 8 times. You can also consult a personal trainer to help you follow a testing protocol that estimates your training load. Once you know how to determine the training load, you can follow the general guidelines found in the table below.

Training Prescription

Research has identified safe, proven prescriptions for each component of muscular fitness. You can fulfill the prescription with calisthenics, weights, or weight machines; you'll get results with hydraulic devices, variable resistance, or free weights. The key to improving strength is to place your muscle under tension for a sufficient amount of time (repetitions and sets). The way you train should be dictated by your level of muscular fitness and how you intend to use the muscles you train. If you have not trained with weights before, use 60 percent of maximal strength (i.e., of your 1-repetition maximum, or 1RM). As you improve your strength, you might increase to 80 percent RM (see the table below). Training is specific in terms of angle, range of motion, and even velocity of contractions. Train the muscles and movements you are anxious to improve.

Muscular Fitness Prescriptions

Component	% max*	RM**	Sets	Recovery***	Days/wk
Strength	70–80%	8–12	1–3	2–3 min	2–3
Muscular endurance	50–70%	15–25	2–3	1 min	2–3

As you gain experience, you may need to increase weight and decrease reps to achieve these goals.

*% max = percent maximum strength: If you can lift 40 pounds, use 20 for endurance (50 percent).

**RM = repetition maximum, the most repetitions you can do with the weight. When you can do more than 12 (or 25) repetitions, it is time to increase the resistance.

***Recovery = minutes between sets.

For example, if you want to train for strength, you should do each exercise using a level of weight that you can lift only 8 to 12 times (8–12RM). You would select an exercise and lift the weight or perform the exercise 8 to 12 times, rest for 2 to 3 minutes, lift it 8 to 12 times again, rest for 2 to 3 minutes, and lift it 8 to 12 times again. Then you would move on to the next exercise and follow the same pattern. You should use resistance training only 2 or 3 days a week. Your muscles need a day between workouts in order to recover.

As you become more experienced, you can

➤ increase the number of sets for strength,

➤ increase weight and decrease reps to improve strength (for instance, using 3 to 8RM),

➤ add more muscular endurance training by increasing the number of reps and sets, and

➤ train muscles more specifically for activity or sport, especially with free weights or sport-specific devices, such as a swim bench for swimming or cord/harness devices for golf, tennis, and softball.

Selection of Exercises

In addition to vital stretching and core training exercises, select strength or muscular endurance exercises to improve your performance in a sport or activity.

improve your performance

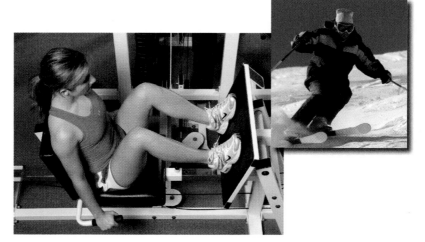

Leg press.

Leg Strength and Endurance ▲

For example, if you are a serious cyclist, your performance and enjoyment will be enhanced if you improve your leg strength and muscular endurance. You will be able to climb bigger hills, push higher gears, and go faster—and still feel less fatigue at the end of the day. Improved leg strength and endurance will also help hikers climb hills and alpine skiers descend them safely. Although training is specific, if you participate in a number of activities, preparation for one will contribute to performance in the others if they use the same muscles in similar ways. Resistance training can improve your performance in cycling, hiking, and skiing, and each activity helps you maintain fitness for the others.

Arm and Shoulder Endurance ▶

Train for arm and shoulder endurance in order to improve your
swimming, cross-country skiing,
or paddling—or all three.

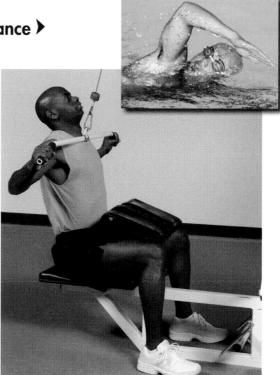

Pull-down.

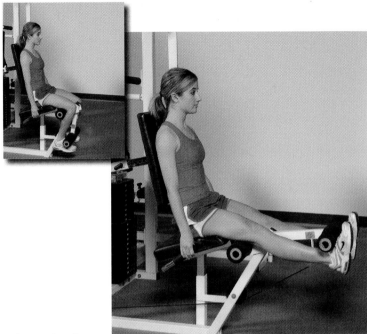

Leg extension.

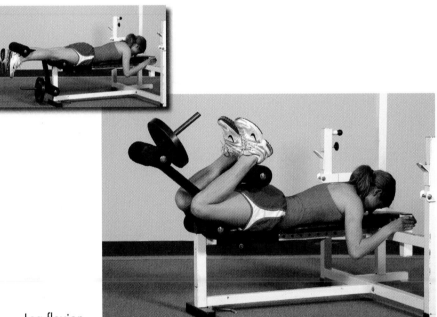

Leg flexion.

Balance in Opposing Muscle Groups ▲

To achieve balance in muscle groups, you may have to train opposing muscles. For example, you should establish and maintain a 3-to-2 strength ratio in your quadriceps and hamstring muscles in order to reduce imbalance and risk of injury. Thus, if you are training your quad muscles, you should balance that training with hamstring work.

Upper-Body Training ▶

If you engage in upper-body activities, you may need to do additional upper-body core training in order to ensure effective power transfer from your trunk to your arms.

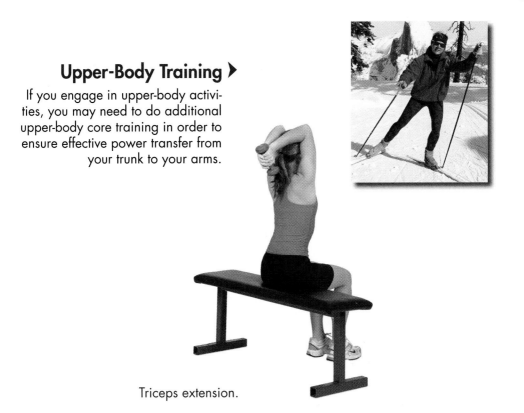

Triceps extension.

Remember Specificity ▼

Remember that training is specific. Once you have developed a list of 8 to 10 exercises, begin the program. Plan to substitute some new lifts every 8 weeks to continue progress and avoid boredom. If you don't have access to a fitness center, you can work out at home. For your upper body, do chin-ups, push-ups, or bench dips.

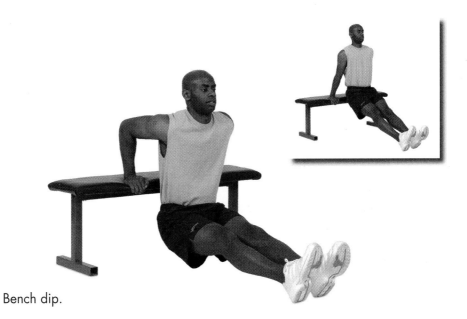

Bench dip.

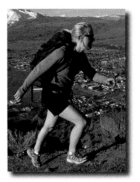

To develop leg strength and endurance, you can wear a weighted vest or pack and climb stairs, repeatedly step up to and down from a bench, or walk up hills. Half knee bends will also help your legs.

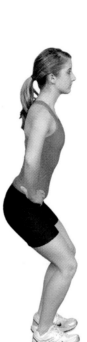

Half knee bend.

Once you get the hang of things, vary your program: Schedule light, moderate, and hard days and weeks of training. For example, do 15RM on Monday, 12RM on Wednesday, and 8RM on Friday.

Following are instructions for some additional resistance training exercises. I have shown some with dumbbells and resistance bands, and you can progress to doing them on exercise machines or with free weights.

Back: Seated Row With Resistance Band ▼

Sit on the floor with your knees slightly bent, and then evenly wrap the resistance band around the insteps of your feet. Sit up straight with your torso perpendicular to the floor. Using a closed grip (thumbs wrapped around the handles), hold onto the handles with your elbows fully extended, your arms about parallel to the floor, and your palms facing each other. The resistance band should be nearly taut (not stretched); if not, take up the slack by wrapping the resistance band farther around your feet.

Pull the handles toward your chest or upper abdomen. Keep your torso upright and your knees in the same slightly bent position. Touch your hands to the sides of your torso. Allow your elbows to slowly extend back to the starting position.

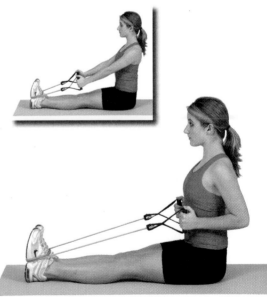

Calves: Heel Raise ❯

You can do this exercise on the floor or on the edge of a stair step. Stand with your hands at your sides or on your hips (hold onto the railing if using stairs). Your feet should be close together and flat on the floor. If you are on a stair step, the weight of the balls of your feet should be on the edge of the step. Rise on your toes 20 to 40 times. For added difficulty, wear a loaded pack.

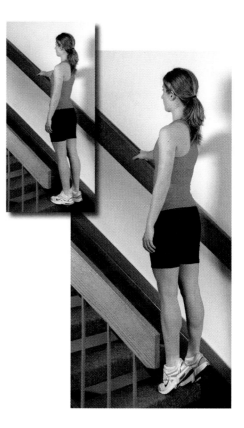

Hips and Thighs: Forward Lunge ▼

At first, the lunge can be done without any weights. Once you learn the technique, you can add light weights in your hands at your sides. Stand straight with your hands on your hips or at your sides. Take an exaggerated step forward; your foot should land on the floor and point straight ahead or slightly inward. Slowly bend your front leg. Allow your rear leg to bend slightly, and then lower your rear leg toward the floor. Your lead leg will be flexed at about 90 degrees, and the lower part of it should be perpendicular to the floor. Shift your balance toward your front leg and push off the floor, shifting your balance to your rear leg. Bring your lead foot back to a position next to your rear leg. Stand tall. Pause. Then alternate lead legs.

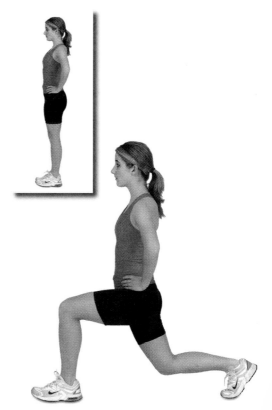

Hips and Thighs: Lunge Jump ▶

Stand with one foot a step ahead of the other. Slowly bend your front leg until your front thigh is at a 90-degree angle to your lower leg. Then immediately jump straight up, extending your knees. Switch the position of your feet on the way down, land, lunge forward with the opposite leg, and jump again. Perform 15 to 25 repetitions. Start gently and increase numbers and intensity slowly.

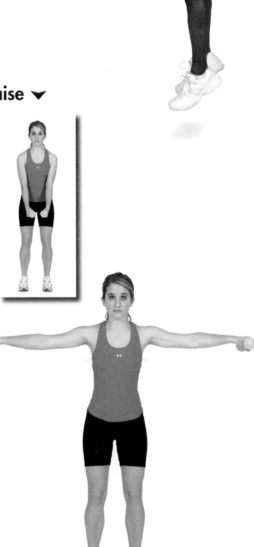

Shoulders: Dumbbell Lateral Raise ▼

Stand with your feet shoulder-width apart and slightly bend your knees. Keep your shoulders back and your eyes focused ahead. Hold two dumbbells at the fronts of your thighs; position the dumbbells so that your palms face each other. Your elbows should remain slightly flexed throughout this exercise, more than is shown in the photos.

Raise the dumbbells up and out to each side; lift both your elbows and your upper arms simultaneously. Keep your upper body straight, your knees slightly bent, and your feet flat. Raise the dumbbells until your arms are almost level with your shoulders and approximately parallel to the floor. At the highest position, your elbows and upper arms will be raised slightly above your forearms and hands. Keeping your knees slightly bent, your feet flat on the floor, and your eyes focused ahead, allow the dumbbells to lower slowly back to the starting position.

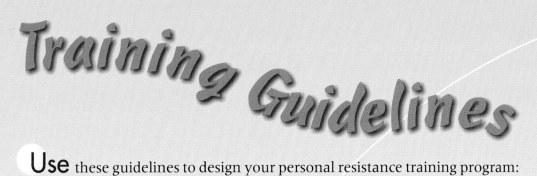

Training Guidelines

Use these guidelines to design your personal resistance training program:

➤ Select 8 to 10 exercises that meet your training goals.

➤ Go easy at first by using lighter weights and fewer sets. Begin with 15RM to 25RM, and then gradually increase the load to 10RM.

➤ Exhale during the lift and inhale as you lower the weight. Do not hold your breath during a lift; doing so can cause several problems, some of them potentially severe. Breath-holding can cause a marked increase in your blood pressure and make your heart work much harder. It restricts both the return of blood to your heart and the flow of blood in your coronary arteries. As a result, your heart gets less oxygen just when it needs more—a dangerous situation, especially for older, untrained individuals. In addition, severe breath-holding can increase intra-abdominal pressure to the point of causing a hernia.

➤ When using free weights, always work with a companion.

➤ When training for strength, allow 2 to 3 minutes of recovery time between sets of the same exercise; when training for muscular endurance, allow 1 to 2 minutes.

➤ Begin with two training sessions per week. After several weeks, move to three sessions per week (you will make optimal progress with three sessions).

➤ Train every other day (e.g., Monday, Wednesday, and Friday) and be sure to eat sufficient protein (e.g., milk or nuts), including 15 grams within 2 hours after training.

➤ Keep records of your progress (see the sample training log on page 184). Test for maximum strength (or endurance) every month, and record your body weight and important dimensions, such as chest, waist, and biceps size.

Muscular Fitness Log

Date	Sit-up	Leg press	Pull-down	OTHER EXERCISES				

Date	Body weight	Waist	Chest	OTHER MEASUREMENTS				

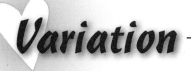

Variation

Experienced lifters use a process that varies training load in order to allow time for recovery. One approach is to make the first week easy, the second harder, the third even harder, and the fourth somewhat easier in order to allow for recovery. If you are training to improve your performance in a sport, you can train for strength in the off-season and for muscular endurance in the preseason. Vary your program, but remember to schedule easier days and weeks in order to allow for recovery. Since progress begins to plateau after 2 months, it helps to change the program every 8 weeks—or whenever your progress plateaus or you get bored.

Designing Specific Programs

You have a lot to think about when designing your own muscular fitness program. The key is to not get too complicated. Think about the activity you want to improve, identify the muscles that the activity involves, and then identify exercises that will help you gain strength, muscular endurance, or flexibility in those muscles. I offer three sample muscular fitness programs on the following pages. The first is a program that you can use if you are just starting out and have no idea what to do. It is a general, all-around muscular fitness program for beginners. The other two sample training programs are geared toward getting a person ready for a several-day backpacking trip. Notice that one uses calisthenics and the other uses resistance training exercises that involve weights. You can accomplish your goals in a variety of ways, whether or not you have access to weight training equipment.

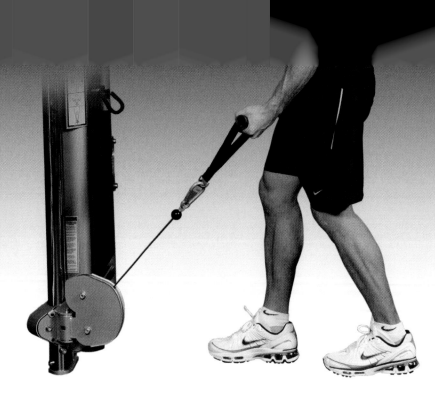

Muscular Fitness Program for Beginners

Train on Monday, Wednesday, and Friday

Type of training	Exercise
Warm-up	Calisthenics
	Brisk walking
	Jogging
Static and dynamic stretching	You select
Core training	Abdominals
	Trunk
Legs	Leg press (or knee bends)
	Leg flexion
	Leg extension
	Heel raises
Upper body	Curls
	Bench press (or push-ups)
	Lat pull-down
	Seated row

Begin with one set of 8 to 12RM; increase to 2 sets after 8 weeks and 3 sets after 16 weeks of training. Switch to muscular endurance training (15–25RM) once you have met your strength goals.

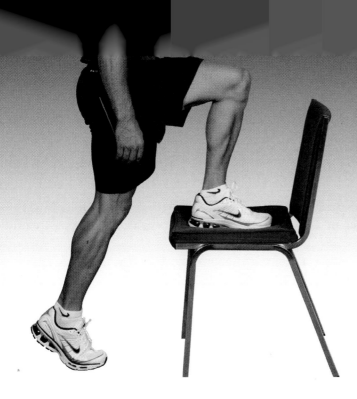

Sample Calisthenics Program for Backpacking Trip on Appalachian Trail

Type of training	Exercise			
Flexibility	Warm up, then do static, contract-and-relax, and dynamic stretches.			
Core training	Do upper and lower abdominal exercises and 2 exercises for the back.			
		Mon	**Wed**	**Fri**
Leg strength and endurance	Knee bends*	2 sets of 20 reps	3 sets of 15 reps**	1 set of 25 reps
	Bench stepping*	2 sets of 20 reps	3 sets of 15RM	1 set of 25RM
Upper body	Push-up***	2 sets RM	3 sets RM	1 set RM
	Chin-up***	2 sets RM	3 sets RM	1 set RM
	Bench dip	2 sets of 20 reps	3 sets of 15 reps**	1 set of 25 reps
	Seated row	2 sets of 20 reps	3 sets of 15 reps	1 set of 25 reps
Cross-training	Mountain biking, stair climbing, and hiking in hills with trekking poles and pack*			

*Start with light pack; add weight as fitness improves. Maximum weight is the load you will carry on the trip (should not exceed 40 to 45 lb or 1/3 of body weight).

**Do slower repetitions at 15RM.

***Can substitute modified push-up or pull-up.

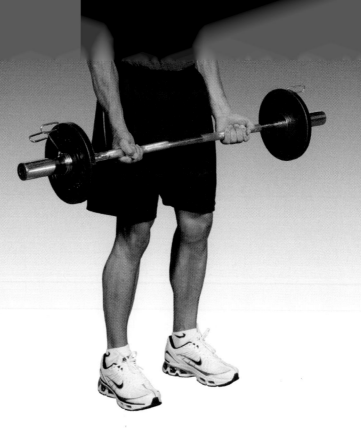

Sample Weight Training Program for Backpacking Trip on Appalachian Trail

Type of training	Exercise	Mon	Wed	Fri
Flexibility	Warm up, then do static, contract-and-relax, and dynamic stretches.			
Core training	Do upper and lower abdominal exercises and 2 exercises for the back.			
Leg strength and power	Leg press	10RM	8RM	12RM
	Leg extension	10RM	8RM	12RM
	Leg flexion	10RM	8RM	12RM
Upper body	Lat pull-down	10RM	8RM	12RM
	Bench press	10RM	8RM	12RM
	Biceps curl	10RM	8RM	12RM
	Triceps extension	10RM	8RM	12RM
	Seated row	10RM	8RM	12RM
Cross-training	Mountain biking, stair climbing, and hiking in hills with trekking poles and pack*			

Start with one set; add another set after 4 weeks and another after 8 weeks.

*Start with light pack; add weight as fitness improves. Maximum weight is the load you will carry on the trip (should not exceed 40 to 45 lb or 1/3 of body weight).

NOW IT'S YOUR TURN... What are your goals? What exercises will help you accomplish those goals? Which of those exercises can you do with the equipment that you have?

Start today!

Design a muscular fitness program and begin to implement it now.

Keys to Muscular Fitness Training

➤ Start easy and make haste slowly.

➤ Warm up and do static and dynamic stretching.

➤ Do core training for back health and performance.

➤ Training is specific; select exercises that meet your training goals.

➤ Schedule light, moderate, and hard days and weeks of training.

➤ Substitute some new lifts every 8 weeks.

➤ Shift to a maintenance program when you are satisfied with your progress.

What's Next?...

You have spent the last few chapters learning how to train for aerobic and muscular fitness. If you haven't developed your own fitness plan based on these guidelines, take time to do so now. Then check out chapter 8 to see how you can improve your health through nutrition and weight control.

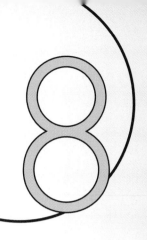

Nutrition and Weight Control

Eat to Live

One must eat to live . . . not live to eat.

~ Molière

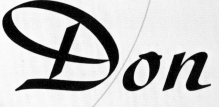

Don

loved basketball, and though he didn't make his college team, he dreamed of becoming a coach. After college, he earned a master's degree in exercise science. Then, to everyone's surprise, he applied for and was appointed to the position of head basketball coach at an inner-city high school. Whereas better-qualified coaching prospects saw the program merely as a perennial cellar dweller, Don saw the job as an opportunity. But his enthusiasm began to wane when preseason practices revealed an emotionally eager but physically listless group of athletes.

...lunch often consisted of an RC and a moon pie

His goal of teaching tough defense and an up-tempo offense seemed unattainable, unless he could find an answer to the team's energy problem.

As he sought to find out why these otherwise healthy young men lacked the endurance to complete a vigorous practice, he discovered that most of them did not eat a good breakfast. On top of that, their lunch often consisted of "an RC and a moon pie" (a cola and a chocolate-covered pastry with cream filling). Don arranged to provide breakfast for the athletes and required them to eat the school lunch. The results were astounding! The players soon had the energy to practice with purpose, and they fought their way to the runner-up spot in the city championship. And, for his part, Don was voted coach of the year.

Nutrition

If you intend to become active, you may need to make modest adjustments in your diet. Since every mile you walk or jog requires at least 100 calories (kilocalories) of energy, you will need to consume sufficient fuel. In particular, you will need to take in enough protein, which, in the form of amino acids, is used to build tissue, produce energy, and develop strength. This section provides basic guidelines to help you eat like an athlete.

Energy

Plants use the sun's energy to grow, after which they often serve as food for animals. We humans get our energy—in the form of carbohydrate, fat, and protein—from plant and animal sources. When you eat and digest food, you absorb fuel into your bloodstream, which transports it to cells throughout your body. You then use enzymes in your metabolic pathways to convert the fuel into high-energy compounds that power your muscles and other cellular activities.

As long as you are alive, you are constantly expending at least some energy. Even if you did nothing at all but lie in bed for 24 hours, you

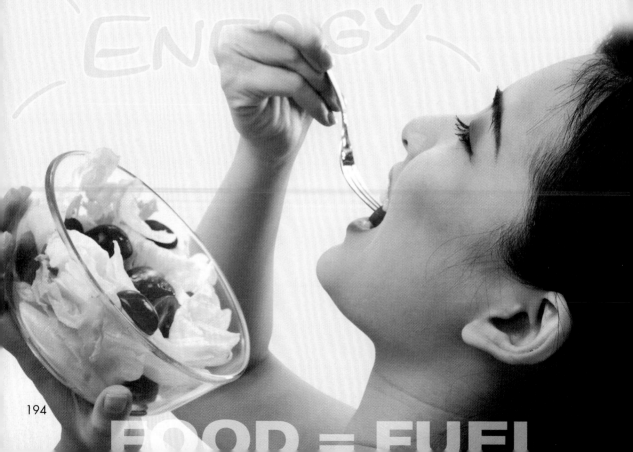

would use about 1,600 calories (if you weighed 154 pounds, or 70 kilograms), which would be used to power your heart and respiratory muscles, fuel your cellular metabolism, and maintain your body temperature. What if you used this time in bed to engage in some hard thinking—tackling a work problem, planning your garden for next spring, or pondering an ethical dilemma you've been avoiding? Perhaps surprisingly, this deep thinking would increase your energy use only slightly. But if you began to move around *physically,* your energy expenditure would increase dramatically. In fact, if you engage in vigorous effort, your caloric expenditure can rocket up from 1.2 calories per minute (at rest) to more than 20 calories per minute. Walking burns about 5 calories per minute, jogging burns about 10, and running burns more than 15. The point here is that physical activity has the greatest effect on your energy needs.

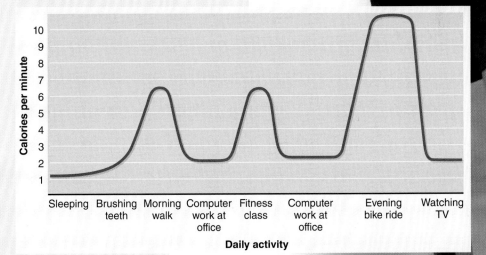

Carbs

Carbohydrate

Carbohydrate, which serves as the major source of energy throughout the world, is available in both simple and complex forms.

SIMPLE SUGARS

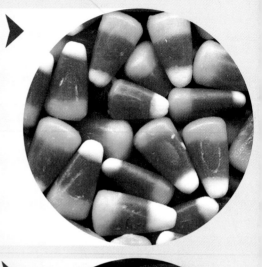

The simple forms contain energy but few nutrients (i.e., vitamins and minerals); they include glucose, fructose, and sucrose (refined sugar, which is composed of molecules of glucose and fructose).

COMPLEX CARBOHYDRATE

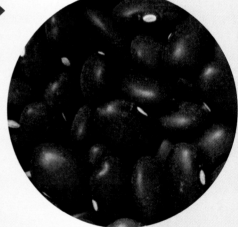

Complex carbohydrate, on the other hand, provides important nutrients and fiber; sources include beans, brown rice, whole-grain products (e.g., bread or pasta), potatoes, and corn. However, despite the ready availability of such healthy foods in the United States, the average American gets half of his or her dietary carbohydrate from concentrated or refined simple sugars, which are packed with so-called "empty calories" (empty in that they lack nutrients).

FRUIT

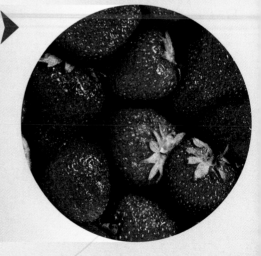

In case you're wondering about fresh fruits, it's true that they contain simple sugars, but they also provide important nutrients.

Even though carbohydrate is important for muscular contractions, your body does not store it in large quantities; as a result, if you are active, you should take in a sizable percentage of each day's calories in the form of complex carbohydrate and fruit. I like to think of a diet for active people as a performance diet, and the table below shows how the performance diet compares with the typical diet. If you are very active, you should get 55 to 60 percent of your daily calories from carbohydrate. This level exceeds the average American diet, in which just 40 to 50 percent of calories come from complex carbohydrate, and it far outstrips the amount consumed by those who choose to partake of whatever low-carbohydrate diet may be currently popular—which is the perfect diet for those who intend to remain sedentary!

Performance Diet

ENERGY SOURCE	PERFORMANCE DIET	TYPICAL DIET
	% of daily calories	% of daily calories
Carbohydrate	55–60	45–50
Fat	25–30	35–40
Protein	15	10–15

Adapted by permission from Sharkey and Gaskill, 2007, p. 213.

Glycemic Index

A food's glycemic index refers to the rate of carbohydrate digestion and its effect on the rise of glucose in your blood. *High*-glycemic foods are digested rapidly and cause a marked rise in your blood sugar; in contrast, due to the fiber or fat content in *low*-glycemic foods, you digest and absorb them more slowly.

HIGH GLYCEMIC INDEX ▸

Foods with a high glycemic index include sugar, honey, white bread, some cereals (those without bran and with high-fructose corn syrup), and baked potatoes.

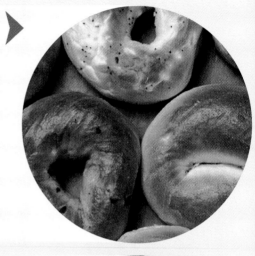

MODERATE GLYCEMIC INDEX ▸

Foods with a moderate glycemic index include pasta, whole-grain breads, rice, corn, oatmeal, bran, and peas.

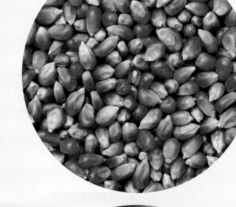

LOW GLYCEMIC INDEX ▸

Foods with a low glycemic index include beans, lentils, many fruits, milk, and yogurt.

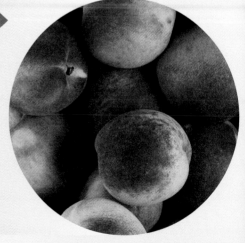

When you eat high-index foods, your blood sugar rises rapidly; you also experience a faster rise in insulin—the hormone responsible for lowering your blood glucose (see the table on the right)—compared with eating low-index foods.

You may be familiar with a condition called insulin resistance, which is often associated with overweight, heart disease, hypertension, a low level of HDL cholesterol (the relatively helpful kind), elevated levels of triglycerides and blood glucose, aging, and inactivity. If you have insulin resistance, you should select foods with a low glycemic index. Even if you have diabetes, you can reduce insulin resistance through weight loss and regular moderate activity.

Should foods with a high glycemic index be avoided altogether? No. They are useful when you want to speed glucose into cells during prolonged exertion. And when you consume a high-glycemic carbohydrate (e.g., potatoes) in a mixed meal, that is, along with fat and protein, you slow the entry of glucose from the high-glycemic food into the blood stream.

Glycemic Index of Common Foods

High-glycemic
Glucose
Sucrose
Cane, maple, and corn syrups
Honey
White breads, including bagels
Potatoes
Cornflakes and most cold cereals
Raisins and bananas
White rice

Moderate-glycemic
Whole-grain breads
Spaghetti
Corn
Oatmeal
Oranges

Low-glycemic
Milk products, including yogurt
Nuts, including peanuts
Legumes (peas and beans)
Apples and peaches

Reprinted by permission from Sharkey and Gaskill, 2007, p. 212.

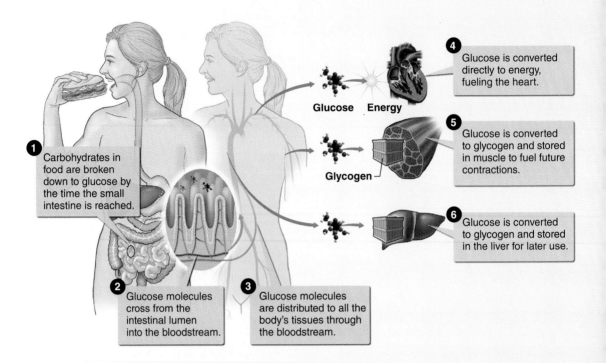

1. Carbohydrates in food are broken down to glucose by the time the small intestine is reached.

2. Glucose molecules cross from the intestinal lumen into the bloodstream.

3. Glucose molecules are distributed to all the body's tissues through the bloodstream.

Glucose   Energy

Glycogen

4. Glucose is converted directly to energy, fueling the heart.

5. Glucose is converted to glycogen and stored in muscle to fuel future contractions.

6. Glucose is converted to glycogen and stored in the liver for later use.

After you eat, your blood takes up sugars and transfers them to cells in your heart, skeletal muscle, and liver, in that order. Your heart, which of course is constantly working, uses the glucose for energy. Your skeletal muscle, in contrast, can store it for later use, and these granules of stored glucose are called muscle glycogen. Your liver also stores glucose as glycogen. Despite these storing functions, taking in *excess* carbohydrate does not give you a supply of "quick energy"; instead, perhaps to your horror, it helps your body conserve fat. The glucose stored in the liver is readily available for your body to transport via your circulatory system and use as needed. Muscle glycogen, however, can be used only by the muscle in which it is stored. Blood glucose is also used by nerves, muscles, or other tissues in need of energy. Thus, when your blood glucose is low (hypoglycemia), you become tired, irritable, confused, and indecisive (see the list of symptoms in the table to the right).

Hypoglycemia Symptoms

Nervousness	Anxiety
Irritability	Confusion
Exhaustion	Rapid pulse
Faintness, dizziness	Muscle pains
Tremor, cold sweat	Indecisiveness
Depression	Lack of coordination
Vertigo	Lack of concentration
Drowsiness	Blurred vision
Headaches	

Reprinted by permission from Sharkey and Gaskill, 2007, p. 312.

Hypoglycemic?

Simple Sugars: The Cause and the Cure

➤ To avoid hypoglycemia, stop eating simple sugars.

➤ If you become hypoglycemic, take in some quickly dissolved high-GI sugar to resolve the symptoms.

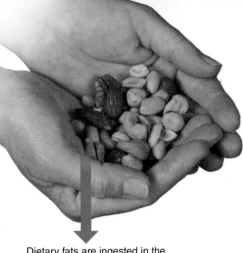

Fat

To most of us, fat is something to avoid. But it isn't all bad. In your diet, fat enhances the taste of food and helps fill you up. In your body, it helps make up your cell membranes and the insulation in your nervous system; it also serves as a precursor for important compounds such as hormones and as a shock absorber for your internal organs. Fat is stored in adipose tissue—loose connective tissue, mainly under your skin but also around your organs—that insulates you and absorbs impacts to your body. Fat can also serve as an efficient fuel for sustained physical activity, especially if you have trained your muscles for endurance. Fat is, in fact, the most efficient way to store energy; it contains 9.3 calories of energy per gram, whereas carbohydrate and protein, respectively, contain 4.1 and 4.3. Dietary fat (the fat you eat) is broken down and absorbed for transport either to your cells for energy or to your adipose tissue for storage. However, dietary fat isn't the only way to acquire this source of energy; excess carbohydrate or protein can also be converted to fat and stored in adipose tissue. Thus, we have many ways to acquire fat but only one good way to remove it—physical activity!

Dietary fats are ingested in the form of triglycerides, which are made up of one glycerol molecule and three fatty acid chains.

Triglyceride

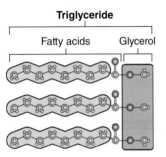

Fatty acids   Glycerol

In the small intestine, triglycerides are split into fatty acids and glycerol and then repackaged back together in a blood-soluble format. This package crosses into the bloodstream.

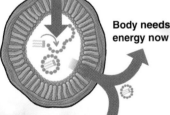

Body needs energy now

Body does not need energy now

Free fatty acids from the triglycerides are delivered to muscle cells and converted to energy.

Later on, when energy is needed, triglycerides are broken down to glycerol and fatty acids, and the fatty acids are delivered to muscle.

Triglycerides are stored whole inside fat cells.

You don't need to eliminate dietary fat; just limit your intake of it. Consuming excess fat is a major cause of overweight and obesity and contributes to heart disease, hypertension, diabetes, some cancers, and other health problems. Fat comes in several forms, including triglycerides and cholesterol. As you may know, saturated fat—found in meat, dairy products, and some oils—is more likely to clog your coronary arteries, since it promotes cholesterol synthesis and the depositing of fat in your arterial walls. As you may *not* know, some otherwise healthful oils can cause the same problem when they are partially hydrogenated, a process that creates trans-fatty acids, thus making otherwise healthy sources of fat dangerous in order to promote a product's shelf life. In contrast, the mono- and polyunsaturated fat found in plants is easily metabolized.

In the performance diet (a diet for active people), you consume 25 percent of each day's calories from fat (no more than 33 percent from saturated fat) and severely reduce your intake of partially hydrogenated fat or trans-fatty acids (see the table on page 197). This recommended portion (25 percent) falls substantially below the 30 to 40 percent that many people currently consume. Happily, your efforts to reduce your fat consumption are likely to be aided by the fact that, as studies show, high fat intake is inversely related to physical activity; in other words, as you increase your level of activity, your fat intake could go down, suggesting a behavioral link between the two (Simoes 1995).

good FAT

Some high-fat foods are actually healthy!

lentils

♥ Nutrition Terminology

triglycerides—Type of fat consisting of three fatty acids and a glycerol molecule. Triglycerides circulate in the blood, and high levels are associated with heart disease and obesity. You can reduce your triglyceride levels by exercising regularly.

cholesterol—Fatty substance found in animal tissue and various foods. Cholesterol is normally synthesized by the liver. Excessive amounts in the blood have been associated with increased risk of heart disease.

saturated fat—Fat, most often of animal origin, that is solid at room temperature. An excess of such fat in the diet is thought to raise blood cholesterol level.

trans-fatty acids—Unsaturated fatty acids produced by partial hydrogenation of vegetable oils. These types of fat are present in hardened vegetable oils, most margarines, commercial baked foods, and many fried foods. An excess in the diet is thought to raise blood cholesterol level.

monounsaturated fat—This type of fat has a higher melting temperature than polyunsaturated fat but a lower one than saturated fat. Monounsaturated fat is usually liquid at room temperature but can turn solid in the refrigerator. Monounsaturated fat is commonly thought of as healthy and may lower your risk of heart disease and stroke.

polyunsaturated fat—Oils made up primarily of polyunsaturated fat are liquid even in the refrigerator. The two main types of polyunsaturated fat are omega-3 and omega-6, which are essential fatty acids, meaning that the body cannot manufacture them.

total fat—Umbrella term including all types of fat.

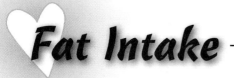

Fat Intake

If you eat 2,000 calories a day and get 25 percent of your calories from fat, you'll get 500 fat calories. Divide that 500 by the 9.3 calories in each gram of fat (500/9.3) and you get 54 grams—the amount of fat you can eat each day. This is far less than the 86 grams you'd eat if you consumed 40 percent of your calories from fat.

Labels on food packages indicate the grams of fat in each serving. Pay attention to this information and stay away from saturated fat and trans fat. Saturated fat should not exceed 33 percent of your daily fat intake.

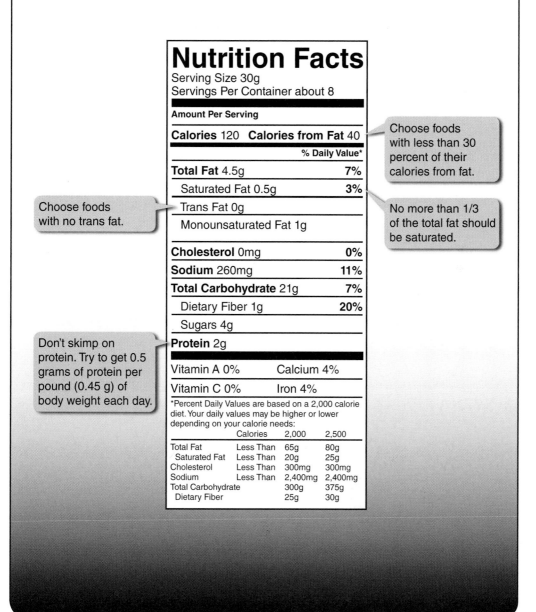

Nutrition Facts

Serving Size 30g
Servings Per Container about 8

Amount Per Serving

Calories 120   **Calories from Fat** 40

% Daily Value*

Total Fat 4.5g	**7%**
Saturated Fat 0.5g	**3%**
Trans Fat 0g	
Monounsaturated Fat 1g	
Cholesterol 0mg	**0%**
Sodium 260mg	**11%**
Total Carbohydrate 21g	**7%**
Dietary Fiber 1g	**20%**
Sugars 4g	
Protein 2g	

Vitamin A 0%	Calcium 4%
Vitamin C 0%	Iron 4%

*Percent Daily Values are based on a 2,000 calorie diet. Your daily values may be higher or lower depending on your calorie needs:

		Calories	2,000	2,500
Total Fat	Less Than		65g	80g
Saturated Fat	Less Than		20g	25g
Cholesterol	Less Than		300mg	300mg
Sodium	Less Than		2,400mg	2,400mg
Total Carbohydrate			300g	375g
Dietary Fiber			25g	30g

Choose foods with less than 30 percent of their calories from fat.

No more than 1/3 of the total fat should be saturated.

Choose foods with no trans fat.

Don't skimp on protein. Try to get 0.5 grams of protein per pound (0.45 g) of body weight each day.

Protein

Protein is crucial to living an active life. When you eat animal or plant protein, the large molecules are broken down into amino acids and absorbed in order to serve as building blocks for constructing cell membranes, muscle tissue, hormones, enzymes, and a variety of other molecules. When you train, you build proteins; specifically, aerobic training builds aerobic enzyme proteins for energy production, whereas strength training builds contractile proteins that are a key to strength.

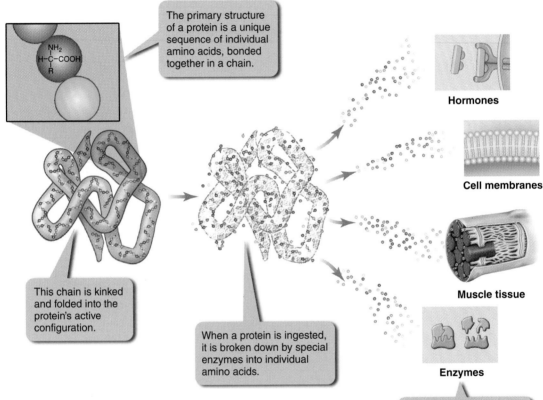

The primary structure of a protein is a unique sequence of individual amino acids, bonded together in a chain.

This chain is kinked and folded into the protein's active configuration.

When a protein is ingested, it is broken down by special enzymes into individual amino acids.

Hormones

Cell membranes

Muscle tissue

Enzymes

The free amino acids can then be used by the body to build a variety of tissues and molecules.

On the performance diet, you consume 15 percent of your daily calories in the form of protein. You can get by on 10 percent if you are moderately active, but 15 percent is better if you are very active or training. For example, 15 percent of 2,000 calories is 300 calories, and 300 divided by 4.3 kilocalories per gram of protein comes out to 70 grams, which amounts to 1 gram per kilogram of weight for a person who weighs 70 kilograms (154 lbs). But there is something even more important than quantity of protein, and that is *quality* of protein. High-quality protein is high in essential amino acids—those that your body cannot create for itself but needs in order to function best. When your body lacks essential amino acids, it is of course unable to construct proteins that require those acids. Animal protein is the best source of essential amino acids (as well as iron and vitamin B_{12}), but you can use proper combinations of plant protein to meet your nutritional needs. If you are a vegetarian or plan to become one, you will need to study the subject (if you haven't already) and learn how to eat a healthful variety of grains, beans, and leafy vegetables.

Protein is not a major source of energy at rest or during exercise; in fact, it is rarely used to meet more than 5 to 10 percent of your energy needs. If, however, you train hard while also dieting to lose weight, your body senses possible starvation and begins to use tissue protein as an energy source. In other words, you lose muscle tissue. To avoid this pitfall and enjoy the benefits you are training for in the first place, ensure that you take in adequate protein and energy. Your best bet is to lose weight slowly—or not at all—during vigorous training.

Salmon = Protein

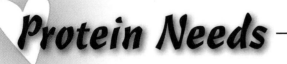

Protein Needs

For the average citizen, the recommended daily intake of protein is 0.8 grams per kilogram of body weight (0.36 g/lb). Endurance athletes, however, need more: 1.2 to 1.4 grams of protein for each kilogram (0.55–0.64 g/lb). And strength athletes need even more: 1.4 to 1.8 grams per kilogram (0.64–0.82 g/lb). These values represent a large increase over the basic recommendation, but you can achieve them through the performance diet (refer back to the table on page 197). For example, if you weigh 70 kilograms (154 lb), multiply 70 kilograms by 1.4 grams (154 lb × 0.64 g) to figure your daily protein needs (98 g). Because each gram of protein yields 4.3 calories, you'll need about 420 calories (98 g × 4.3) of energy from protein. The table below indicates the protein available in some common foods.

Protein in Common Foods

Food	Portion	Protein (g)
Beans	1/2 cup (118 ml)	6–8
Beef	4 ounces (113 g)	20–28
Cheese	1 ounce (28 g)	7
Chicken	3 1/2 ounces (100 g)	24–30
Chili	1 cup (236 ml)	20
Corn	1/2 cup (118 ml)	3
Fish	4 ounces (113 g)	25–30
Hamburger	4 ounces (113 g)	20
Milk	1 cup (236 ml)	9
Peanut butter	1 tablespoon (14 ml)	4
Pizza	1 slice	10

Reprinted by permission from Sharkey and Gaskill, 2007, p. 216.

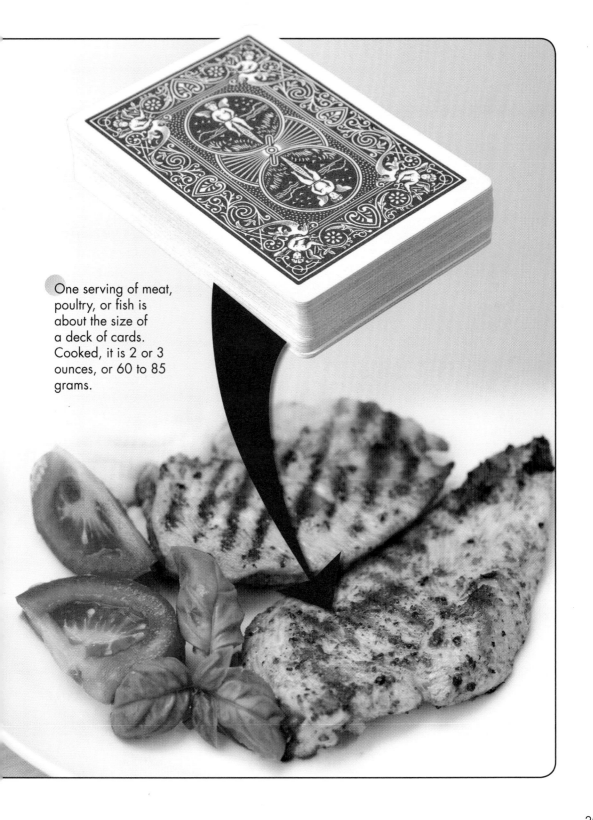

One serving of meat, poultry, or fish is about the size of a deck of cards. Cooked, it is 2 or 3 ounces, or 60 to 85 grams.

Athletes raise their total caloric intake to meet the increased energy needs of training. If you find yourself feeling sluggish or fatigued in your training, increase your intake of good-quality protein (lean meat, skinned poultry, fish, beans, or nuts; see the table on page 208). On the other hand, if you eat more protein than you need, along with fat from animal sources (eggs, meat, fish, poultry, or dairy products), you will promote the storage of fat. Follow the performance diet, and you will have the protein you need, since the high carbohydrate intake spares or conserves your tissue protein during training.

Finally, pay attention not only to the quality and amount of protein you eat but also to the timing of your protein intake. Be sure to eat some of your daily protein within 2 hours after you exercise so that your body can use it to rebuild tissue.

Available Energy

So, how much energy is available in your body, anyway? You have a limited supply of glucose (from carbohydrate) in your blood, but it is needed for brain and nerve metabolism, for which it is the sole energy source. Glucose is also stored as glycogen in your liver (about 80 grams) and in your muscle (15 grams per kilogram [33 g/lb] of muscle). If you could use all of this fuel for exercise, you would have about 1,200 calories, which is about enough to power a 10-mile (16.1 km) run.

Fat is the most abundant source of energy. Young women average over 30 percent body fat; young men average 15 percent. If you weigh 121 pounds (55 kg) and have 25 percent body fat, you have about 30 pounds (14 kg) of fat, which amounts to 105,000 calories (each pound of fat

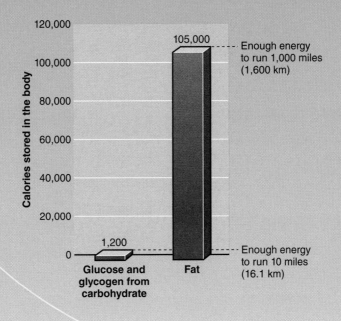

yields 3,500 calories). This is enough fat energy to fuel 1,000 miles (1,600 km) of jogging! If, like most of us, you have more fat than you need, you can benefit from training your body to burn more fat during exercise. You can do so through long-duration exercise sessions, which improve your access to fat stores. With improved aerobic fitness, then, you extend your aerobic endurance dramatically, eliminate the problem of excess fat and body weight, and improve your overall health.

Vitamins and Minerals

We have been discussing carbohydrate, fat, and protein—all of which are macronutrients. Vitamins and minerals, in contrast, are called micronutrients because we need only small amounts of them on a daily basis. Even so, they play essential roles in cell metabolism, immune function, clotting, and other key functions.

Vitamins

If vitamins do not supply energy and are needed only in minute quantities, why do we consider them essential for life? The answer in many cases is that vitamins are coenzymes—the active portion of enzymes that perform specific tasks essential to the chemical

Vitamins

reactions that help your body function properly. For example, vitamin B_1 (thiamine) is a coenzyme that removes carbon dioxide from molecules; without vitamin B_1, the process grinds to a halt, allowing a toxic buildup of compounds in your cells. Deficiency of vitamin B_1 leads to beriberi, a disease characterized by weakness, wasting, nerve damage, and even heart failure.

The small amounts of vitamins that you need are readily available from a variety of foods in a well-balanced diet. Doses that far exceed your daily requirements (megadoses) do not improve bodily function or performance, and they may even be toxic.

Vitamins are classified according to solubility—that is, how well they dissolve in water or fat. B-complex vitamins and vitamin C are water-soluble, and excess water-soluble vitamins are simply flushed away in your urine, meaning that you are unlikely to build up toxic levels but more likely to experience a deficiency. This can occur if you go several days with low intake of a vitamin. In contrast, you ingest the *fat*-soluble vitamins A, D, E, and K when you consume fat, and excess amounts of these vitamins are not flushed away but rather are stored in body tissue; as a result, megadoses can become toxic. Since these vitamins are stored, you are less likely to be deficient in them, unless you are following a very low-fat diet.

FitFact

In most cases, you can get the vitamins and minerals you need from eating a well-balanced diet. Taking doses that exceed daily requirements will not make your body work better.

Vitamins and the Immune System Vitamins perform many functions essential to your health, including the operation of your immune system. You can help your immune system remain healthy by including the following micronutrients in your well-balanced diet:

BETA-CAROTENE

(carrots, sweet potatoes)

stimulates immune system cells
that fight infection

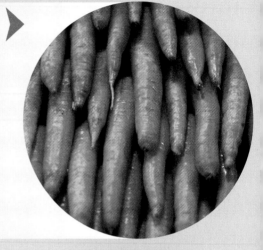

VITAMIN B$_6$

(potatoes, nuts, spinach)

promotes proliferation of
white blood cells

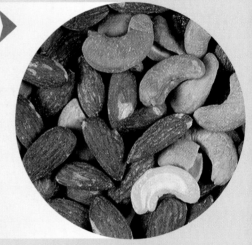

FOLATE

(peas, salmon, romaine lettuce)

increases white blood cell activity

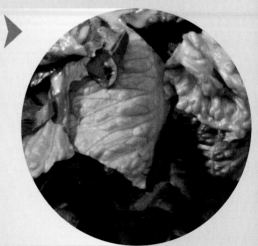

VITAMIN C

(citrus fruits, broccoli, peppers)

an antioxidant that enhances
immune response

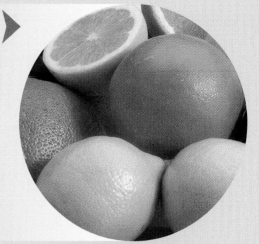

VITAMIN E

(whole grains, wheat germ, vegetable oils)

an antioxidant that
stimulates immune response

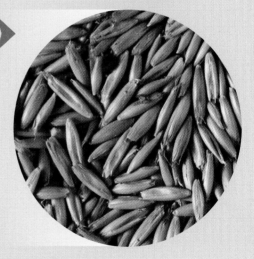

Immune response is also aided by certain minerals and by physical activity. Selenium promotes action against toxic bacteria and is found in tuna, eggs, and whole grains. Zinc promotes wound healing and is found in eggs, whole grains, and oysters. Regular moderate physical activity boosts your immune system, whereas exhaustion and stress impair it, thus opening the door to upper respiratory and other infections.

Antioxidants   Intense exercise produces compounds called free radicals; these harmful molecules can also derive from various other sources, including exposure to air pollution or UV light. Free radicals are highly reactive compounds that can damage your muscle tissue, especially if you are untrained and have limited antioxidant capability. We do have some natural antioxidant protection, but the supply is limited.

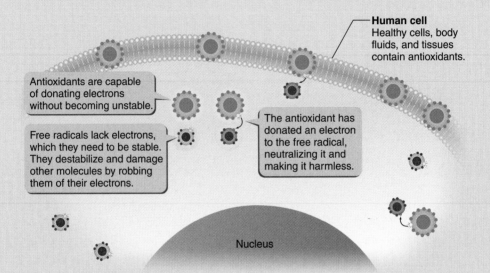

Human cell
Healthy cells, body fluids, and tissues contain antioxidants.

Antioxidants are capable of donating electrons without becoming unstable.

Free radicals lack electrons, which they need to be stable. They destabilize and damage other molecules by robbing them of their electrons.

The antioxidant has donated an electron to the free radical, neutralizing it and making it harmless.

Nucleus

Antioxidants seek out free radicals and bind to them, neutralizing the free radicals so they cannot harm the body.

Fortunately, antioxidant vitamins and regular activity and fitness training have been shown to reduce free radicals' ability to damage your body. Beta-carotene and the vitamins C and E—the so-called antioxidant vitamins—may minimize muscle damage from free radicals and even reduce your risk of heart disease, cancer, and eye disease. In the case of heart disease, the antioxidant vitamins may prevent the deterioration of lipids, which is a step in the artery-clogging process of atherosclerosis.

With all this mind, you should begin—

FitFact

The American Heart Association, the American Cancer Society, and the American Dietetic Association agree.

Scientific data do not justify the use of vitamin supplements to reduce heart disease, cancer, or other health problems.

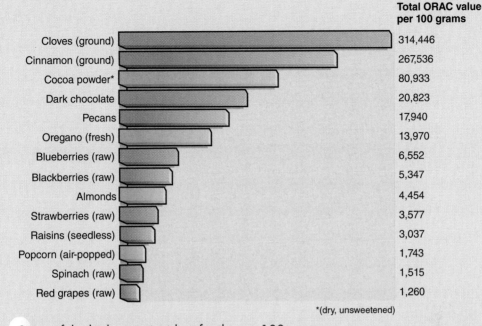

	Total ORAC value per 100 grams
Cloves (ground)	314,446
Cinnamon (ground)	267,536
Cocoa powder*	80,933
Dark chocolate	20,823
Pecans	17,940
Oregano (fresh)	13,970
Blueberries (raw)	6,552
Blackberries (raw)	5,347
Almonds	4,454
Strawberries (raw)	3,577
Raisins (seedless)	3,037
Popcorn (air-popped)	1,743
Spinach (raw)	1,515
Red grapes (raw)	1,260

*(dry, unsweetened)

Some of the highest antioxidant foods, per 100 grams.
Adapted from U.S. Department of Agriculture, 2007.

now—to consume a diet that is rich in natural antioxidants. Taking vitamin supplements is not as effective as consuming the same nutrients in fruits and vegetables; to put it more bluntly, vitamin supplements are not a satisfactory replacement for a well-balanced diet. The vitamins you get from food come with other vitamins, minerals, and trace nutrients that appear to enhance the antioxidant effect. Supplementing with vitamins to achieve the Dietary Reference Intake (DRI) may offer a small margin of safety for those who lose considerable weight during training or refuse to eat nutritious food. (Visit fnic.nal.usda.gov and do a search on "DRI tables.") Otherwise, get your micronutrients by eating a variety of nutritious foods.

Minerals

Ever wonder why your body needs things like iron, zinc, magnesium, and chromium—but definitely not lead? Minerals are vital to various processes within your body: enzyme and cellular activity, hormone production, bone health, muscle and nerve activity, and acid–base balance. Your body needs very small amounts of some minerals (less than 100 milligrams daily) and more of others. You can consume minerals in many food sources, but concentrations are higher in animal tissue and animal products. Like vitamins, minerals are readily available in a well-balanced diet that features a good amount of variety. However, if you cut a major nutrient source from your diet (e.g., meat), problems can arise.

Even though minerals are essential to your health and ability to perform, supplementing with minerals beyond what your body needs is not only unnecessary but could cause side effects. Some minerals are harmless even if consumed in excess, but others can cause diarrhea (magnesium or zinc), high blood pressure (sodium), or cirrhosis (iron). If you have reason to believe that you may be deficient in minerals—for example, if you are training hard while losing weight in order to improve your performance—consider taking a supplement that provides the recommended daily intake for vitamins and minerals. Even in this case, however, remember that supplements do not provide a substitute for good nutrition through diet. For more information on nutrition, see the *Dietary Guidelines for Americans* provided by the U.S. Department of Health and Human Services at www.health.gov/dietaryguidelines.

FitFact

Supplements are not a substitute for good nutrition. Eat nutritious food to live healthier and longer.

Eggs are a good source of zinc, iron, selenium, phosphorous, and iodine.

Weight Control

This section of the chapter addresses what you take in, what you use, and what happens if you eat more than you use: overweight and obesity. In ages past, when the human food supply was unpredictable even for the lucky ones, people could not count on three square meals a day (much less snacks); as a result, the human body learned how to store energy in the form of fat. Today, most of us enjoy access to a dependable and plentiful food supply, but our bodies still store energy even though the need for doing so is gone. This contradiction has created a problem in that two-thirds of the U.S. population is overweight or obese (Centers for Disease Control and Prevention). We deposit lots of calories into our body's energy account but generally withdraw smaller amounts, and our energy balance grows and grows. The following discussion should help you balance your energy and control your weight.

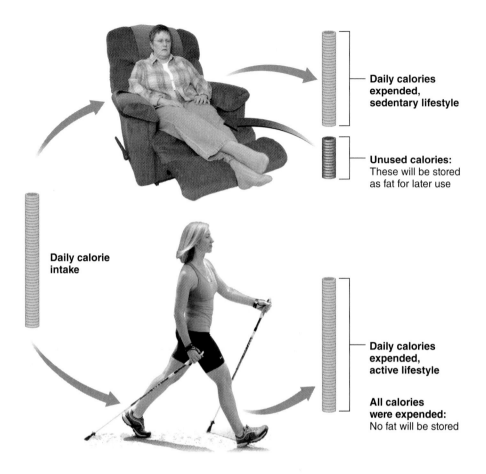

Daily calories expended, sedentary lifestyle

Unused calories: These will be stored as fat for later use

Daily calorie intake

Daily calories expended, active lifestyle

All calories were expended: No fat will be stored

Energy Intake

I have discussed the fact that your body takes in energy in the form of carbohydrate, fat, and protein. Once you store energy, it remains in your body until it is used. But just where is it kept?

Carbohydrate is stored in clumps of glucose called glycogen in your liver and muscles. The portion stored in your liver acts as a reserve that helps maintain your level of blood glucose, which is the essential energy source for your brain and nervous tissue. Muscle glycogen, on the other hand, is the fuel that powers high-intensity contractions, and you cannot sustain that kind of work when this fuel supply gets depleted.

Fat is stored in your adipose tissue, around organs (visceral fat), and in your muscles. Your body uses fat stored in your muscles as energy for contractions, especially when you engage in activity of lower intensity but longer duration. When muscle fat is depleted, your body can mobilize fat from adipose tissue and transport it by means of your circulatory system to power your working muscles.

When you eat protein, the amino acids it contains are used to build proteins in your body. Of the energy you use in doing an activity, only a small portion (5 to 10 percent) comes from tissue protein. Your body will, however, break down muscle to get protein for energy if you are on a starvation diet.

Energy Expenditure

As you may recall from earlier discussion, your energy use jumps any-time you move your body around. Energy is also needed when you eat, because the processes of digestion and absorption themselves must be fueled. Still, it is overt physical activity that has the greatest effect on your energy expenditure.

The predominant source of energy for light- and moderate-intensity exercise is fat. When you exercise at high intensity, however, your pri-mary fuel is carbohydrate in the form of muscle glycogen; your use of carbohydrate as fuel is also somewhat higher if you exercise moderately after eating a high-carbohydrate meal. If you exercise continuously for several hours, the relative contribution of each fuel changes throughout that period. For example, at 75 percent of $\dot{V}O_2$max, the contribution of muscle glycogen drops from almost 50 percent to near 0 upon depletion of the supply. Meanwhile, the role of blood glucose increases from 5 to 40 percent, but when your liver glycogen supply declines, blood glucose

EXPENDITURE

itself falls precipitously. Thus, the contribution of fat from adipose tissue increases throughout prolonged exercise, rising from 25 to 50 percent after several hours. Runners "hit the wall" when muscle and liver glycogen and blood glucose become depleted.

Your energy expenditure depends in part, of course, on your body size. The more you weigh, the more calories you will use for a given activity. To understand how this works, see the figure on page 49 and the energy expenditure chart in the appendix. For example, if you weigh 140 pounds (64 kg) and bicycle moderately hard (10 mph), you will burn about 4.5 calories per minute. But if you weigh 160 pounds (73 kg) and do the same activity, you'll burn about 5.1 calories per minute.

Physical Activity and Weight Control

Weight loss is a matter of energy balance: Eat less, burn more, or, for best results, do both. To eat less, use a smaller plate, reduce fat and oil, and eat fruit for dessert. Here are your options for losing weight:

➤ **Go on a diet.** Many diets show early success due to the loss of water previously stored with carbohydrate. However, you might not like the long-term consequences. See the discussion on dieting on page 224.

WEIGHT LOSS OPTIONS

Dieting?

For many people, dieting causes weight gain. That's right—weight *gain*. When you diet, your body becomes more fuel efficient and your metabolic rate declines. As a result, even more dieting or exercise is required in order to reduce excess weight. During this cycle, your weight loss slows, and you regain weight three times faster. Eventually, your body will maintain weight on a low-calorie diet that actually makes it harder for you to lose weight and easier for you to regain it.

How does this happen? When you diet, your body uses protein for energy, which means that you lose muscle protein with each dieting cycle. And when you lose muscle—the furnace that burns excess calories—you reduce your capacity to burn calories, regardless of whether you are at rest or doing exercise. Thus, each time you diet to lose weight, you lose lean tissue and must therefore decrease your caloric intake in order to avoid subsequent weight gain. If you return to your former eating habits, you increase your weight and fat *above* previous levels. As a result, the only way to minimize the loss of lean tissue while dieting is to exercise. In fact, if you do enough exercise, you can reverse the drop in your metabolic rate and increase your lean tissue, thereby easing the problem of weight control.

The Diet–Weight Gain Cycle

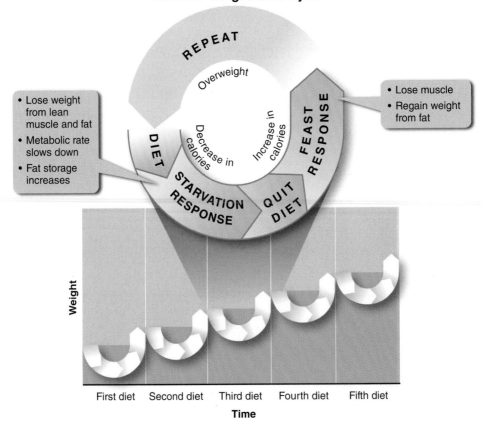

REPEAT

Overweight

Decrease in calories

Increase in calories

DIET

STARVATION RESPONSE

QUIT DIET

FEAST RESPONSE

- Lose weight from lean muscle and fat
- Metabolic rate slows down
- Fat storage increases

- Lose muscle
- Regain weight from fat

Weight

First diet　Second diet　Third diet　Fourth diet　Fifth diet

Time

➤ **Take a pill.** For a hefty price, you get modest weight loss—so long as you continue to take the pill. When you stop, however, the weight returns. And, of course, you will experience side effects while taking the pill.

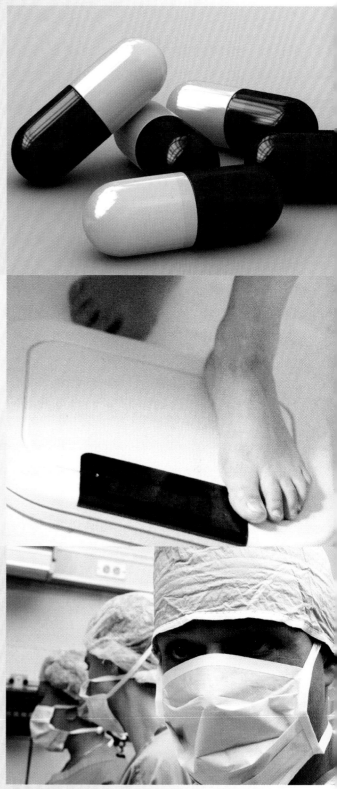

➤ **Fast.** The ultimate way to restrict caloric intake is, of course, to fast. It is guaranteed to result in dramatic weight loss, as much as a pound (0.45 kg) a day, but it also carries risks, especially if you do it for an extended period, and it makes it hard for you to perform vigorous exercise. An occasional day of fasting will do no harm under ordinary circumstances, but you should avoid extended periods of fasting.

➤ **Get surgery.** If you are morbidly obese—more than 100 pounds (45 kg) above normal weight—then surgery to form a smaller stomach may be prescribed. It seems to work, at least for a while, but it is extremely expensive and risky, and it requires lifelong changes in your eating behavior.

➤ **Eat less and exercise more.** The ideal approach is to eat fewer calories and burn more with physical activity. Doing so burns fat even as it conserves protein. Improving your fitness leads to additional benefits that improve your health and performance:

- Increased caloric expenditure
- Increased use of fat
- Reduced blood lipids (cholesterol and triglycerides)
- Increased lean tissue (muscle)

Control your weight with moderate food intake and enough regular exercise to achieve energy balance. Some types of exercise are better than others for weight control. As you know, we shift from fat to carbohydrate metabolism as exercise becomes more vigorous. Therefore, if you want to burn excess fat, do more moderate exercise. In addition, because extremely vigorous activity cannot be sustained for very long, your total caloric expenditure may not be great. Remember, too, that fat use increases over time (more fat is burned after 30 minutes of exercise), and that you can continue light or moderate activity for hours without undue fatigue, thereby achieving significant metabolism of fat and expenditure of calories.

Incidentally, while we are on the subject of fat metabolism, the best time to exercise for weight control may be in the morning, before breakfast. The reason? You are more likely to burn fat after an overnight fast. So if you are interested in fat metabolism and weight control, try morning exercise. If that approach doesn't suit your biological clock, however, don't give up. Exercise always burns calories, so it always contributes to weight control.

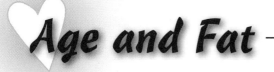

Age and Fat

With each decade above age 25, your body loses about 4 percent of its metabolically active cells, so you naturally burn fewer calories as you age. As a result, if your diet remains relatively unchanged over a 10-year period, you will probably gain weight. This reality means that you'll need to either exercise more or eat less in order to maintain a desirable weight. Not only that, but the loss of metabolically active cells with age usually means a decline in *lean* body weight, including muscle, and an *increase* in body fat. Being regularly physically active will help you counteract these changes.

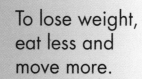

FitFact

To lose weight, eat less and move more.

A Practical Weight Loss Program

With two-thirds of the United States population overweight or obese, you might think that losing weight is extremely difficult, but this is true only if you ignore the question of energy balance. To lose weight, you must burn more calories than you consume. You might have your own proof of this from a day when you were physically busy and didn't eat your typical amount of food—your pants probably fit a little looser at the end of that day.

The National Weight Control Registry (NWCR) has been investigating long-term successful weight loss maintenance since 1994. This group looks at the characteristics of people who have succeeded at long-term weight loss. The NWCR is tracking over 5,000 individuals who have lost significant amounts of weight and kept it off for long periods of time. Although there is variety in how NWCR members keep the weight off, most report that they maintain a low-calorie, low-fat diet and do high

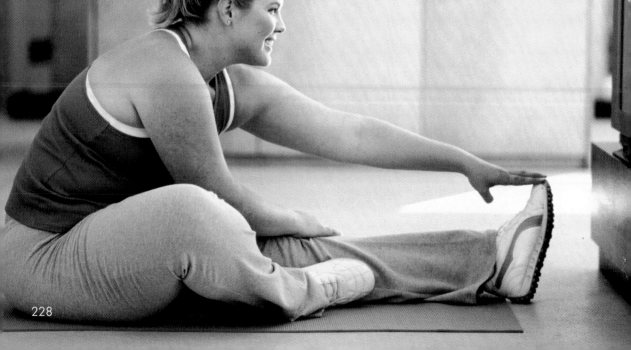

levels of activity. They share some other common characteristics:

- ➤ 78 percent eat breakfast every day.
- ➤ 75 percent weigh themselves at least once a week.
- ➤ 62 percent watch less than 10 hours of TV per week.
- ➤ 90 percent exercise, on average, about 1 hour per day.

Other medically monitored studies have proven that moderate caloric restriction and moderate physical activity can produce a 25 percent weight loss without adverse health effects (Keys et al. 1950).

So how should you proceed?

1. Increase your aerobic and muscular fitness exercise. Do a moderately long workout at midweek and a long one on the weekend.

2. Do not diet; diets are associated with weight gain.

3. Reduce your caloric intake by cutting back on food portions (use a smaller plate, e.g., 9 inches in diameter) and reducing your intake of high-fat and low-nutrient foods.

4. Eat breakfast every day.

5. Weigh yourself at least once a week.

6. Watch less TV.

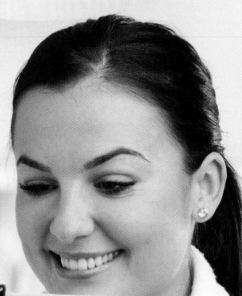

Your goal for weight loss should be to lose 1 pound (0.45 kg) per week but never to lose more than 2 pounds (0.9 kg) in a given week. If you are very overweight, with a body mass index above 30, you may need to add behavioral therapy to your exercise and caloric restriction plan. This approach involves learning to behave in new ways, such as keeping a food diary, using positive self-talk, and rewarding yourself for good behavior. For a detailed weight control program—including tips for moderate caloric intake and energy expenditure, along with a behavioral modification program—see *Fitness and Health* (Sharkey and Gaskill 2007). You might also look into healthy eating programs offered in your community or online. One such program is Healthy Eating Every Day (see a description on the Web site for Active Living Partners at www.ActiveLiving.info).

Keys to Nutrition and Weight Control

➤ If you are very active, consume 55 to 60 percent of each day's calories in the form of complex carbohydrate (beans, brown rice, corn, potatoes, or whole-grain products) and fruit.

➤ Limit your fat intake and avoid saturated fat and trans fat.

➤ Eat sufficient high-quality protein (15 percent of your daily caloric intake) to meet your protein needs during training.

➤ Achieve weight control by balancing your caloric intake with your caloric expenditure.

➤ Since metabolic rate declines with age, you will have to eat less, engage in more activity, or do both in order to maintain a healthy weight.

➤ Remember that dieting often leads to future weight gain, especially when it is done without physical activity.

What's Next?...

You've learned about healthy eating and the importance of balancing the food you eat (calories in) with your physical activities (calories out). In chapter 9, we'll review how much activity you need and what to do if you have health issues or exercise problems.

Health Issues and Exercise Tips

Overcoming Hurdles

All mankind is divided into three classes: those that are immovable, those that are movable, and those that move.

~ Arab proverb

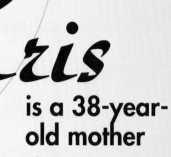

Kris

is a 38-year-old mother

of two boys who is recovering from a mastectomy and chemotherapy. At first, she fatigued easily, and she was mildly depressed for several months and unable to keep up with her two sons.

Her husband picked up the slack and urged her to join him for evening walks. In time, she began to recover, mentally and physically, and she decided to set some activity goals to motivate herself to work toward further recovery. A family conference led to a decision to spend their summer vacation hiking the trails of Glacier National Park. With her doctor's approval and with advice from a fitness instructor, Kris began preparing for the trip by undertaking focused aerobic and muscular fitness training. By the time summer rolled around, she was able to keep up with her husband and sons as they hiked to Avalanche, Hidden, and Iceberg lakes and explored other popular trails in the park. Since then, Kris has formed a women's hiking group that provides its members with emotional and physical support.

What Activities Have Purpose for You?

It helps to have an activity goal in mind, similar to Kris in our opening story. You might start by simply meeting the recommendations for activity, but soon into your ventures, you will need something more compelling to keep you going. First, let's refresh your memory of the basic guidelines for the amount of activity you should get.

You may remember from chapter 1 that the *2008 Physical Activity Guidelines for Americans*, published by the U.S. Department of Health and Human Services (www.health.gov/paguidelines/), calls for adults to do 2 hours and 30 minutes a week of moderate-intensity—or 1 hour and 15 minutes a week of vigorous-intensity—aerobic physical activity, or an equivalent combination of moderate- and vigorous-intensity aerobic physical activity. You can gain additional health benefits by increasing to 5 hours a week of moderate-intensity aerobic physical activity, or 2 hours and 30 minutes a week of vigorous-intensity physical activity, or an equivalent combination of both. Adults should also perform muscle-strengthening activities that involve all major muscle groups on 2 or more days per week. For more on these guidelines, see chapter 1, page 9.

FitFact

You should be physically active for at least 30 minutes on 5 days a week in activities that you enjoy.

Choose a Meaningful Activity

As you think about how to implement these exercise recommendations, remember to choose activities that are meaningful to you. More than 80 percent of the United States population is not active enough, and 67 percent is overweight or obese (Centers for Disease Control and Prevention). When individuals join a fitness class, half of them drop out within weeks. Apparently, the class failed to meet their needs. The same is true at fitness clubs: Dropouts usually exceed the number of long-term participants. However, if you engage in an activity that has purpose or meaning for you, you are much more likely to stick with the program.

Dog owners, for example, rarely miss a walk, even in bad weather. Those who heat their home with wood seldom fail to split, stack, and carry wood. Create meaning by setting goals: Train for a long hike, a bike ride, a paddling trip, or a vigorous vacation. Prepare for cross-country or downhill skiing, tennis, or golf; vow to walk the golf course as long as you are able.

What are your activity goals, and what activities would be meaningful to you?

Health Issues

Many people rely on their doctor to take care of their health; unfortunately, this approach doesn't work. No doctor can make you live more healthily—that is, lose weight, eat better, stop smoking, wear a seat belt, or exercise regularly. Yet these simple habits—one's lifestyle—account for more than half of all disease and death; in fact, they affect health and disease more than the practice of medicine does. Having said that, it's true that medical tests and periodic visits to the physician are important. You can use community or employee health or wellness programs for blood

Healthy Habits

Lose
weight

Eat
better

Stop smoking

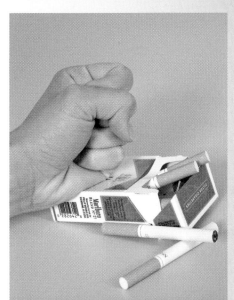

Wear a seat belt

Exercise regularly

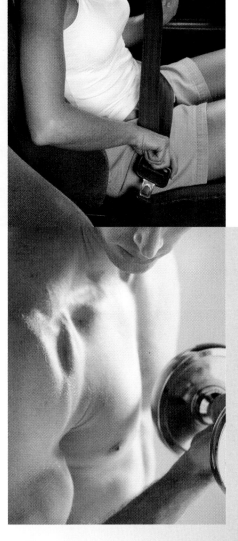

tests, blood pressure checks, and other exams; and, of course, if you have symptoms or are concerned about your health, then by all means see your physician. But do you need an annual medical examination? Many researchers question the need for an annual preventive health exam, citing the high costs as well as the facts that the majority of preventive care occurs outside of physical exams and most patients were seen by physicians for another reason during the same year (Mehrotra, Zaslavsky, and Ayanian 2007). I see my physician annually to discuss any questions and to renew prescriptions. Every so often, he persuades me to take an important test (e.g., to have a colonoscopy). Here's another question: Should you see the physician before you begin an exercise program?

Preexercise Medical Examination?

In chapter 1, you had the opportunity to take a health screening questionnaire to help you identify whether you need to see your physician before engaging in vigorous activity. If you didn't complete the questionnaire then, take a few minutes to do it now.

Should you see a doctor before increasing your physical activity? Eminent physician and exercise scientist Dr. Per Olaf Åstrand (Åstrand and Rodahl 1970) had this to say:

> As a general rule, moderate activity is less harmful to the health than inactivity. You could also put it this way: A medical examination is more urgent for those who plan to remain inactive than for those who intend to get into good physical shape!

If you are free of symptoms and follow a sensible program to gradually transition into new or more exercise, then living actively is certain to enhance your health rather than threaten it. However, if you have any of the following circumstances, then you should consider getting a medical examination beforehand: you have been sedentary, are concerned about your health, have one or more risk factors for heart disease (e.g., hypertension, elevated cholesterol, smoking, or inactivity), or are over 45 years of age for men or over 55 for women and plan to start a vigorous exercise program.

If you have known cardiac, pulmonary, or metabolic disease—or if you have symptoms or are over 45 years old for men or 55 for women—then the American Heart Association (AHA) and the American College of Sports Medicine (ACSM) recommend that you get a medical exam, including a progressive ECG-monitored exercise test (or stress test) *before* you engage in vigorous exercise.

Risks of Activity

The risks of activity and fitness training range from minor musculoskeletal problems to major coronary events. The benefits of activity increase rapidly at first but eventually plateau. Risks, on the other hand, rise slowly at first, and then more rapidly at higher levels of activity. For most of us, then, it seems prudent to maximize benefits and minimize risks by engaging in a level of activity associated with enhanced health—that is, regular moderate activity.

FitFact

It is generally more risky to your health to be inactive than to start exercising.

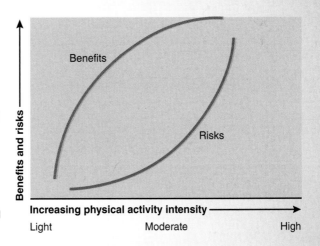

Relationships of benefits and risks with levels of physical activity. You can maximize benefits and minimize risks by doing regular moderate activity.

Reprinted by permission from Powell and Paffenbarger, 1985, p. 123.

Warning Signs

As you engage in physical activity, be aware of these warning signs.

WARNING SIGNS

WARNING SIGNS

STOP Signs If you experience any of these symptoms, *even once*, stop exercising and consult your physician before resuming.

➤ **Abnormal heart action.** This may take the form of an irregular pulse; fluttering, pumping, or palpitations in your chest or throat; a sudden burst of rapid heartbeats; or a very slow pulse (either during or after exercise) that was moderate just a moment earlier.

➤ **Pain or pressure in the middle of your chest or in your arm or throat.** This can occur during or after exercise.

➤ **Dizziness, lightheadedness, sudden loss of coordination, confusion, cold sweat, glassy stare, pallor, blueness, or fainting.** Stop the exercise—do not try to cool down—and lie with your feet elevated, or sit and put your head down between your legs, until your symptoms pass.

YIELD Signs Try the suggested remedy; if it doesn't help, consult a doctor.

➤ **Persistent rapid heart action.** It is normal for your heart rate to increase with exercise intensity. But if your heart beats too fast when you are exercising vigorously and continues to beat fast for 5 to 10 minutes afterward, you should adjust your workout. To correct the problem, lower your exercise intensity (in terms of heart rate) to a comfortable level, then increase it slowly over a period of weeks. If the problem persists, consult a physician.

➤ **Flare-up of bone or joint conditions.** Rest and resume exercise when the condition subsides. If the usual remedies (e.g., ice) do not help, see your doctor.

CAUTION Signs These problems can usually be remedied without medical consultation, though you may wish to report them to your doctor at your next visit.

➤ **Nausea or vomiting after exercise.** Wait at least 2 to 3 hours after eating before you exercise; also avoid extreme heat, exercise less vigorously, and take a longer cool-down period.

➤ **Extreme breathlessness lasting more than 10 minutes after you stop exercise.** Exercise less vigorously, at a level where you can hold a conversation (per the talk test). See your doctor if the problem persists.

➤ **Prolonged fatigue.** If you remain tired for 24 or more hours after exercising or have insomnia related to physical activity, lower your exercise intensity, then increase it gradually over a period of weeks.

➤ **Side stitch.** Lean forward while sitting and tighten your abdominal muscles or exhale through pursed lips.

Exercise Problems

FitFact

If you have not been active before, you might run into a few problems when you first begin to exercise. As a first step, try to prevent these problems—preventing them is easier and better than treating them. Then, if a problem does arise, treat both the symptom and the cause. For example, if your ankle hurts, go ahead and ice it, but then find out why it hurts (e.g., wrong shoes for your activity) and correct the problem for good.

Make every effort to *prevent* exercise problems so you won't need to deal with them.

Blisters

Blisters are minor burns caused by friction. You can prevent them by taking proper measures before you exercise: Wear properly fitted shoes, use appropriate socks (double-layer or tube), and apply a lubricant (e.g., Bag Balm) to hot spots. If you are in the midst of a prolonged effort (e.g., backcountry hiking or skiing), take action at the first sign of trouble by covering the area with duct tape—yes, duct tape. A good tape job can last several days. You can treat more advanced cases with a sterilized hollow needle: Release the fluid, treat the area with an antiseptic, circle it with a foam rubber donut, and then carry on.

Muscle Soreness

You may experience what is called delayed-onset muscle soreness (DOMS) about 24 hours after undertaking a new or more vigorous exercise. It may derive from swelling or microscopic tears in your muscle or connective tissue. If you ease into a sport gradually, you will minimize this type of soreness, and you

soreness

can make subsequent activity less uncomfortable by warming up and doing mild stretches. You can also reduce pain by massaging the affected area. Fortunately, DOMS is a short-lived inconvenience that protects you against further discomfort for several months—or until you start a new sport, but you can take comfort in the fact that this too will pass in relatively short order.

Muscle Cramp

A cramp is a powerful involuntary contraction. Your nervous system usually tells your muscles when to contract and relax, but this normal control sometimes fails, and when it does you will certainly feel the result! You can achieve immediate relief by stretching the cramped muscle and massaging it (always toward the heart), but the underlying cause will remain. Dehydration and high temperatures seem to make muscles susceptible to cramps, and we know that the chemistry of contraction and relaxation involves sodium, potassium, and calcium. Therefore, if you are going to be active in hot weather, make sure you take care of your body's need for fluid and electrolyte replacement. While water is fine for an hour or less of activity, our studies of wildland firefighters at the University

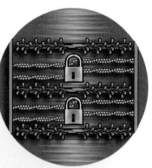

In a muscle cramp, muscle filaments lock into a contracted position, causing pain when you attempt to lengthen or stretch the muscle.

of Montana indicate that popular sports drinks that contain water, electrolytes (sodium and potassium), and carbohydrate enhance prolonged performance in hot conditions. The carbohydrate provides energy and minimizes the effects of prolonged exertion on immune function.

Bone Bruise

Active people, especially hikers and joggers, sometimes get painful bruises on their feet. In some cases, this type of injury is not just a garden-variety, soft-tissue bruise but rather an injury to the bone itself. Bone bruises are less serious than fractures, but they can take a long time to heal (a bad one can last for weeks). You can avoid such bruises by using high-quality footwear and watching where you place your feet, for example, taking care not to step hard on sharp rock edges while hiking. Bone bruises result from repetitive impacts, and you can reduce those shocks by using shoes with cushioned inner soles and gel or air soles. While you recover, you can use ice to reduce discomfort; you can also see if a little extra padding in your shoe allows you to engage in some activity. Finally, take a look at your shoes; a bone bruise may indicate that it's time to replace them.

Ankle Sprain

Treat an ankle sprain through the RICES approach (see the list below). Ice your ankle immediately, preferably in a bucket of ice water, and continue to ice it for 20 minutes several times a day for 3 to 4 days. Rest and elevate your ankle between icing sessions, and use a wrap to stabilize it and maintain compression. One way to minimize recurrences is to wear high-top shoes whenever possible.

Rest

Ice

Compression

Elevation

Stabilization

Muscle Pull

You should never ignore a pulling sensation in your calf or hamstring. You can treat a minor pull with rest and ice. In addition, for a calf pull, try a gel heel cup; for a hamstring pull, an elastic sleeve may let you get active again more quickly. In either case, return to activity cautiously—a serious pull can take weeks to heal. To prevent muscle pulls, take time to warm up, perform focused stretching, and purchase good footwear.

Area of pull

Use focused stretching, such as this calf stretch, to help prevent muscle pulls, which can take weeks to heal.

Shin Pain

Pain on the front of your shinbones is called shin splints and can be caused by muscle spasm or by inflammation of the muscle, its membrane, or the bone. For relief, use rest, compression wraps, deep massage (toward your heart), and anti-inflammatory medications (e.g., ibuprofen). To prevent shin splints, transition gradually into training, steer clear of hard running surfaces, reverse your direction occasionally if you run on a short indoor track, use a heel-to-toe footstrike, perform resistance exercises, and remember to stretch.

Knee Pain

Researchers have found that running does not harm healthy knees. Problem is, many of us run on less than healthy knees! Some of us even run on knees that are already afflicted with osteoarthritis. Cumulative physical stress adversely affects knees, and handling heavy loads (at work or in sport) increases your risk of knee osteoarthritis.

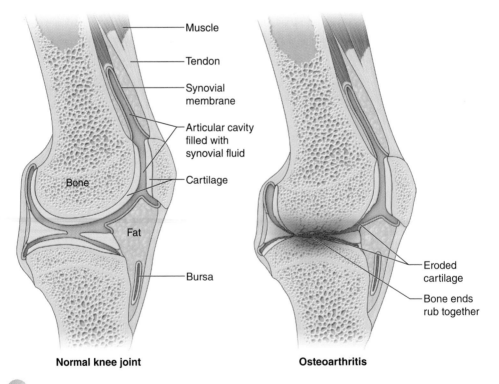

Normal knee joint   Osteoarthritis

In osteoarthritis, you lose the cushioning of cartilage at your joints, and your bones start to rub together.

Exercising With Arthritic Knees

Thanks to a high school football injury, I have an arthritic knee (the cartilage was removed more than 40 years ago). Nonetheless, I have been able to continue hiking and running. How? The answer is threefold: weight training to stabilize my thigh and hamstring muscles; cycling to gently add strength and endurance; and use of nonsteroidal anti-inflammatory drugs (NSAIDs) such as aspirin and ibuprofen to reduce inflammation and discomfort. If I overdo it with the degenerative knee, I rest, ice, and use a bit more of the NSAID until it settles back down.

If you experience knee trouble, attend not only to the symptom but also to the cause. Here are two ideas: First, try new shoes or arch supports. In addition, if you run a lot, try alternating between two pairs of shoes—one with padding for sore feet, the other with a flexible sole for sore legs. If these approaches don't do the trick, consult an athletic trainer or podiatrist who specializes in sports medicine and ask whether foot supports (orthotics) make sense for you; these inserts can correct pronation and reduce some knee pain. Try store-bought orthotics before you invest in custom inserts.

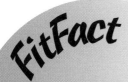

FitFact

For injuries or other problems, correct the cause while you treat the symptom.

Who Should You See for an Activity Injury?

Who should you consult when you experience an activity- or sport-related injury? A physician? A specialist (orthopedist)? I go to the sports medicine specialist with the most experience in sport-injury prevention, diagnosis, and treatment—an athletic trainer. Unfortunately, most folks don't have access to a trainer, so they go to one doctor and then another, thus running up a medical bill. You may be able to find a trainer, however, at a sports medicine clinic, high school, or local college. If not—and if friends and the World Wide Web don't provide an answer—then your next best bet is to see a physical therapist, who will either recommend a treatment or refer you to an appropriate medical specialist. If you do see a specialist, be sure to leave with a treatment plan in hand. My favorite orthopedic surgeon is closely associated with a physical therapy center. When I exit his office, I enter the center. Whatever the problem—from a sprained ankle to a knee replacement—early ambulation is the secret to success in rehabilitation!

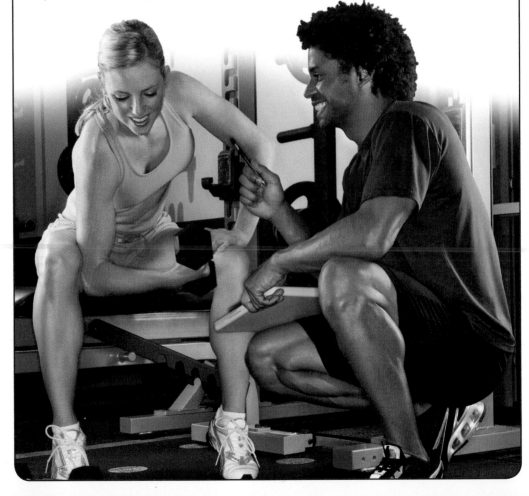

Special Considerations

If you have a special exercise concern or limitation, this section is for you. It briefly summarizes several issues, and if you are interested in additional information you can consult specific books (see www.humankinetics. com), the Web, local community service agencies, or your physician.

Older Adults

As you age, your need for muscular fitness increases. If you are older, be sure to do exercises that enable you to develop and maintain muscular strength and endurance.

In particular, take steps now to increase your strength to necessary levels before loss of strength undercuts your independence.

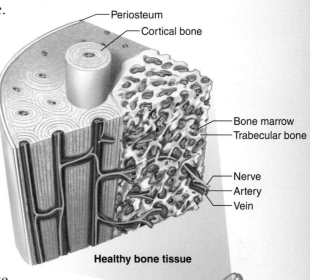

Healthy bone tissue

Women

The advice and prescriptions presented in this book work for both men and women. If you are a woman, however, you should consider several additional issues. Girls who have yet to experience puberty need to know that high-volume, vigorous training before puberty may delay the onset of the menstrual cycle. On the positive side, such a delay is associated with a lower risk of cancers of the breast and reproductive system. At the same time, bone-related problems can result either

Strength training and other weightbearing activity, such as walking, improves bone density, which is particularly beneficial for women, who often get osteoporosis with age.

251

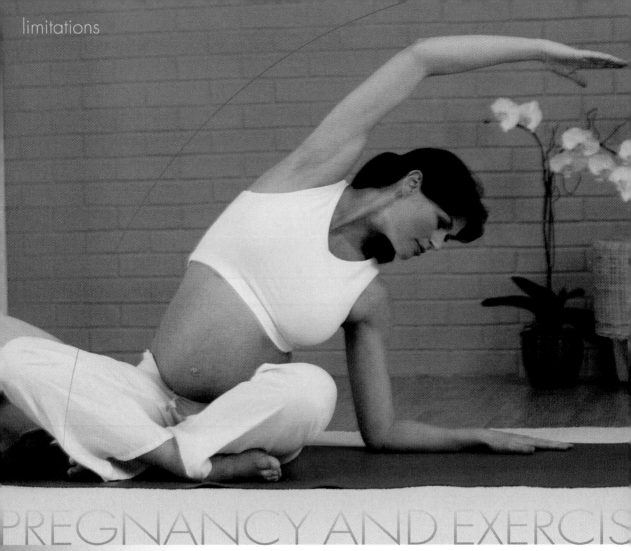

PREGNANCY AND EXERCIS

from a long delay in the onset of menstruation or from amenorrhea (suppression of menstruation) due to excessive aerobic endurance training in young women; specifically, these problems may include reduced bone mineral content, stress fractures, and increased risk for osteoporosis. On the other hand, strength training not only increases muscle mass and strength but also strengthens bones.

If you are pregnant, you may continue your exercise program with your physician's approval. There are several reasonable precautions: Most doctors recommend that you step away from high-impact aerobics, keep your exercise heart rate below 140 beats per minute, and avoid prolonged exposure to high temperatures during activity. If you are postmenopausal, you should participate in activities that minimize the progress of osteoporosis; specifically, do exercise that moderately stresses the muscles and bones of your upper body and your legs. And no matter your age, you need to be aware of women's special nutritional needs—be sure to include enough calcium and iron in your diet.

Disease or Disability

Every condition involves its own restrictions—and its own potential. These days, people with disabilities participate in a wide variety of physical activities and compete as high as the international level, but only after establishing control over their conditions. They ski, kayak, and do just about anything, and more opportunities are becoming available every day. People with diabetes, for example, compete in all kinds of sports and have even topped Mount Everest. Wheelchair athletes compete in marathons, play basketball, and go fishing. People with multiple sclerosis respond better to moderate activities, such as swimming. For more information, contact a recreation department, a community service organization, or the National Center on Physical Activity and Disability, which maintains a wonderful (and free) electronic newsletter and Web site (www.ncpad.org).

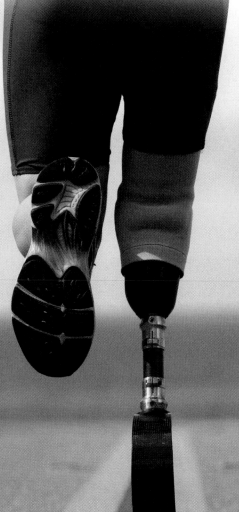

REACH YOUR POTENTIAL

Work and Travel

Neither work nor travel should be an excuse for missing out on exercise. Find a way to exercise at work. Wear walking shoes so you can walk to or from work, during breaks, or at lunchtime. Take the stairs instead of the elevator. Use company facilities or join a gym. The same goes for travel. Carry exercise gear on the road. Walk whenever possible, especially in airports. Walk as you discuss business. Select a hotel with a fitness center, and use it every day.

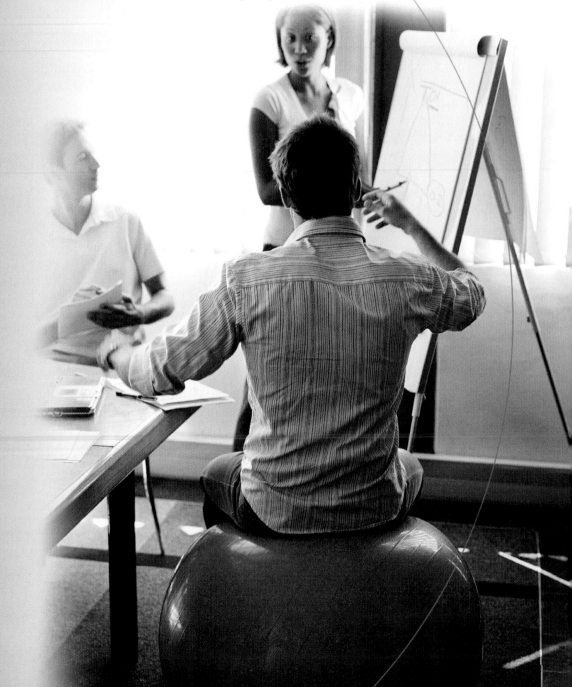

Fitness Clubs

People join fitness clubs for advice, access to equipment, and social reasons. To differentiate between a good fitness club and a bad one—between an effective program with qualified staff and a fly-by-night organization—you should visit the club for a tour and a free introductory session. Is the facility clean and well equipped? Does the equipment meet your needs? Are the patrons satisfied? (Do they encourage you to join?) You should also ask about the staff members' qualifications and credentials. Do they have degrees in the field from reputable institutions? Do they have experience? Are they certified? Are they all trained in emergency response?

The American College of Sports Medicine (ACSM) certifies health and fitness instructors and program directors who meet educational and experience standards and successfully complete a rigorous test. More generally, ACSM publishes standards for health clubs and offers a brochure to help you evaluate a club. To request a copy of the brochure, write to ACSM at PO Box 1440, Indianapolis, IN 46206-1440, or visit the group's Web site at www.acsm.org. You can also use the checklist on page 256 to evaluate fitness facilities as you shop around.

If you decide to join a club, avoid long-term contracts. Also be wary of discounts and other high-pressure tactics; they may be signs of a failing business or of high member turnover. Sign up for a few months or until you are absolutely certain that the club meets your needs. Then, if time permits, become active in an advisory group that works with management to maintain and upgrade staff qualifications, facilities, and equipment.

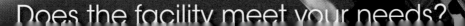

Does the facility meet your needs?

Checklist for Evaluating Fitness Facilities

Answer yes or no to each question for each facility.

Question	Facility A	Facility B	Facility C
Convenience. Is the facility convenient? Is it near home or work?			
Hours. Do the hours of operation fit your needs?			
Parking. Is the parking adequate?			
Facilities and equipment. Does the club have the facilities (e.g., pool, racquetball courts, or aerobics studio) and equipment (e.g., free weights, weight machines, or aerobic machines) that you want to use?			
Space. Is the space ample in the showers, locker rooms, and fitness rooms and on the courts and tracks?			
Availability. Are activity spaces and equipment available at the time when you would plan to use them?			
Physical condition. Are the facility and its equipment clean, neat, well maintained, and in good working order?			
Air quality. Are the temperature, humidity, and ventilation controlled and comfortable at peak times?			
Programs. Does the facility provide comprehensive fitness programming (aerobic, strength, and flexibility training) as well as sports activities? Does the facility offer any special programming in which you are interested (e.g., for older adults or pregnant women)?			
Special services. Does the facility provide comprehensive health and fitness services (fitness assessments, goals and action plans, physical therapy, arthritis therapy, cardiac rehabilitation, weight loss programs, and nutrition counseling)?			
Staff. Are staff experienced, well qualified, and certified by recognized agencies such as the American Red Cross (CPR and first aid), the American College of Sports Medicine (ACSM), the American Council on Exercise, and the Cooper Institute? Are the staff members healthy role models? Are they friendly and supportive? Are personal trainers available?			
Supportive systems. Are activities available to encourage adherence (recognition programs, challenges and contests, monitoring systems, or recreational leagues)?			
Safety and security. Are safety and security practices emphasized (written policies and procedures and appropriate signage)?			
Cost. Is the membership fee affordable for you? Are there any hidden costs? Must you sign a contract?			
Add other considerations here:			

Adapted by permission from Ettinger, Wright, and Blair, 2006, pp. 123-124.

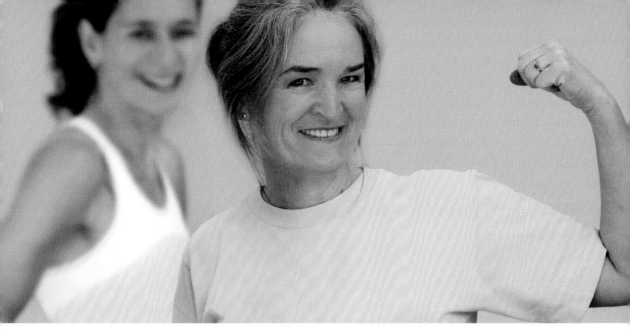

Keys to Health Issues and Exercise Tips

➤ Childhood is the best time to become active; the next best time is now.

➤ Begin now and strive to meet the physical activity guidelines—at the very least, 30 minutes of moderate-intensity exercise most days of the week.

➤ Select meaningful activities—those with a purpose.

➤ If you become ill or injured, seek treatment; then return to activity as soon as possible.

➤ Find a way to exercise at work (e.g., take walking shoes).

➤ Plan to be active when you travel (e.g., select a hotel with a fitness center).

➤ Join a fitness club if it meets your needs.

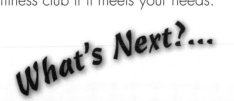

In this chapter, you considered how to make activity more meaningful for you. You also learned whether you need to see a doctor before stepping up your activity level and things to watch for when you become active, including tips for resolving exercise problems. Turn the page to chapter 10 to learn facts and fallacies of fitness.

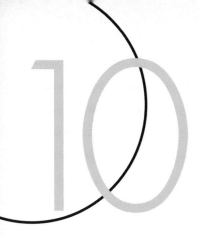

Fitness Facts and Fallacies

What's the Truth?

He who cannot rest, cannot work; he who cannot let go, cannot hold on; he who cannot find footing, cannot go forward.

~ Harry Emerson Fosdick

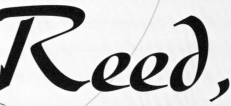

Reed,

a musician,

joined a fitness club to help him pursue a New Year's resolution to become more fit. After a few days of aimless effort, he decided to engage the services of a personal trainer. Tim was a lean, muscular trainer who promised rapid results. After a week of working with Reed on a moderate lifting program, Tim said it was time to crank it up to a higher level. So Reed did more sets and more repetitions—and often found himself suffering complete fatigue of a muscle group.

He was promised rapid results...

His muscles were sore, and he experienced decreased ability to lift and a feeling of lassitude. The intense training made it difficult for Reed to work, so he took a break and then sought the services of another trainer who better understood his needs. In following Tim's overly intense approach to training, Reed had in fact been approaching a condition called exertional rhabdomyolysis, in which damage to muscle membranes allows cellular components to leak out and cause kidney damage. Now, after weeks of moderate muscular and aerobic endurance training, Reed can complete a musical gig and then engage in after-hours improvisations.

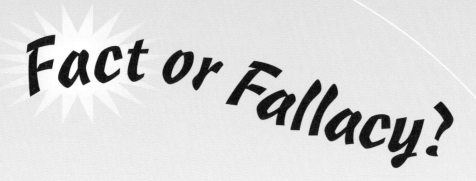

Fact or Fallacy?

This chapter considers the facts and some of the fallacies that abound in the world of physical activity. It also describes how facts are properly established in order to help you become a better consumer of information about fitness and health.

Facts

How does a hypothesis or theory become a fact? Carefully planned and controlled studies help us separate fact from fiction. Exercise physiologists conduct many types of studies in order to understand the immediate and long-term effects of exercise and training (see the table on the following page). In status or comparison studies, we are able to determine differences between groups, such as athletes and nonathletes. Such studies can show differences, but they don't prove why athletes are stronger or faster (chances are that their heredity and environment predispose them to become successful in a particular sport). Another type of study—the correlation study— looks at the relationship of one factor (e.g., a particular training method) to another factor (e.g., performance). These studies are used to show the relationship of training volume (e.g., miles or kilometers per week) to performance in swimming, running, and other events; they do not, however, prove the need for high-volume training. Why not? The reason

Types of Research Studies

Type of research	How it's done	Proves cause and effect?
Status	**Compares groups** 	No
Correlation	**Determines relationships among variables** Time Performance Distance	No
Experimental	**Manipulates variables** Control group Experimental group	Yes

Adapted by permission from Sharkey and Gaskill, 2006, p. 8.

is that a relationship does not prove cause and effect. For example, a swimmer may be successful *in spite of* heavy training, or because he or she was able to survive the ordeal while others became run down.

The type of study that allows us to draw cause-and-effect conclusions is called an experimental study. Subjects are pretested, randomly assigned to either experimental or control groups, monitored for progress during carefully controlled training, and posttested at the end of the experiment. A physiologist can use an experimental study to determine the effects of a particular training method with more confidence. For example, if an experimental training technique improves performance more than the traditional approach does, the result is significant if statistical analysis indicates less than a very small probability (less than 5 percent) that the outcome is due to chance. The result is considered *highly* significant if analysis indicates less than a 1 percent probability (i.e., less than 1 chance in 100) that the results were due to chance. When the preponderance of studies agree on the

FitFact

In research, a relationship does not prove cause and effect.

effect of a type of training, the status of that technique changes from hypothesis or theory to proven fact.

Of the three types of research, only experimental studies allow us to draw a cause-and-effect conclusion. Experimental studies involve manipulating a variable, such as the number of sets of resistance training, to determine whether that variable can be used to improve an important measure, such as strength.

You don't need to conduct research or read research journals in order to answer questions about physical activity. That is my job. I've distilled the essence of the findings in order to present the information in simple terms. In the future, you can use books, magazines, and the Internet to increase your understanding of physical activity and fitness. But be careful; as you will see in this chapter, the world is full of untested "facts." Advertisements and infomercials often promote a product with testimonials from athletes or attractive models. Some even claim that the product or technique has been proven effective in scientific or clinical studies. That is seldom true. If you are interested in a product, ask to see the studies.

The rest of this chapter presents some facts and principles about exercise and training—facts based on numerous studies and field observations. Then it lists some fallacies and misconceptions that have little or no basis in medical or scientific research.

Training Principles

This section introduces a dozen important facts and principles that you should act on in order to avoid illness and injury and make steady progress in your training.

Readiness—You need to be physically and psychologically ready to train in physical activity. Physical readiness requires that your body have sufficient nutrition and rest to be able to benefit from training.

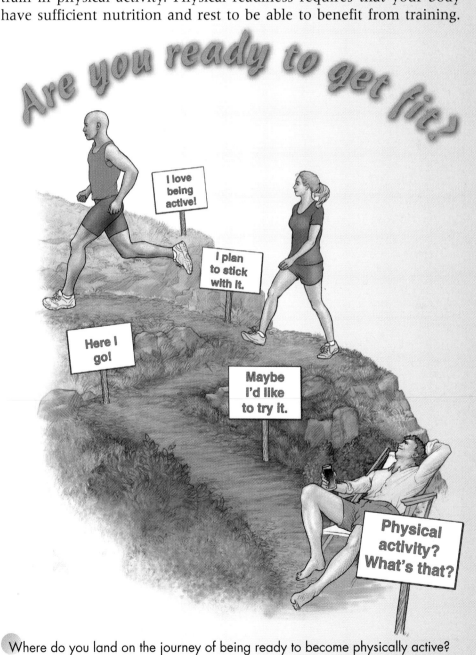

Where do you land on the journey of being ready to become physically active?

Psychological readiness refers to your commitment to train, to delay gratification, and to make the sacrifices involved in sustained training.

Adaptation—Training brings on subtle changes as your body adapts to added demands. Daily changes are so small that you will not notice them, but if you progress patiently for weeks and then months, you will see measurable adaptations, including improved respiration and heart function; improved muscular endurance, strength, and power; and tougher bones, ligaments, tendons, and connective tissue.

Individual response—Different people respond differently to the same training. Reasons include heredity, maturity, nutrition, rest and sleep, level of fitness, environmental influences, illness or injury, and motivation.

Overload—If you want to achieve the desired adaptations in your body, you must train in a way that places demands on your system. Training must exceed your typical daily demand or load; as you adapt and get stronger, you must increase the load. Your rate of improvement hinges on three factors, which you can remember with the help of the acronym FIT: frequency, intensity, and time.

Progression—To achieve adaptations using the overload principle, you must train according to the principle of progression. If you increase your training load too quickly, your body will be unable to adapt; instead, it will break down. At the same time, progression does not imply inexorable increase without time for recovery. Your body needs periods of rest in which the desired adaptations take place. *Make haste slowly!* The principle of progression also has other implications: Your training should progress from general to specific and from quantity to quality. Athletes often taper training before a major competition so they will be rested and ready to go. You should too.

Specificity—In order to achieve desired results, you must train specifically for those results. Specific training brings specific results. You won't get much stronger through aerobic endurance training, and you won't improve your aerobic endurance very much through strength training. Put another way, cycling is not the best preparation for running, or vice versa. Your performance will improve most when your training is specific to the activity in which you are interested.

Of course, any rule or principle can be taken to an extreme, and specificity does not mean that you should avoid training opposite or adjacent muscles. For example, some cycling may be good for a runner, since it will provide muscle balance, train adjacent fibers, and offer some relief from the pounding of running.

FitFact

In order to improve, you must train more frequently, more intensely, or for more time.

Cross-Training

Cross-training is a way to avoid overuse injuries. It allows addicted athletes to train hard every day with little risk of overuse or repetitive trauma injury. Some people extol the virtue of training a variety of muscle groups, as in swimming, cycling, and running. Triathletes train for all three disciplines, and they also do sport-specific weight training to enhance performance. Cross-training allows athletes and fitness enthusiasts the option of training more than they could in a single sport; it also enables them to achieve balance in their training.

But does cross-training provide special performance benefits? Probably not. Specificity is still the best rule to follow if you want to improve in a sport. Swimming, for example, will not improve your performance in running or cycling. Cross-training does not raise your performance above the level that you can attain through sport-specific training. Activities that use similar muscles may contribute somewhat to performance, but not to the same degree as do increases in specific training. Of course, cross-training is an absolute necessity if you are preparing for a multiple-discipline event, and it is a great way to remain active and fit as you grow older!

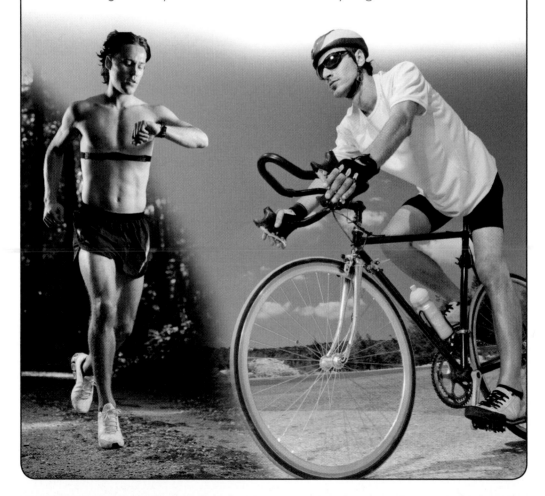

Variation—In order to avoid boredom and maintain your interest, you should vary your training program. Your body adapts as desired when you follow work with rest and when you follow the hard with the easy. When possible, conduct workouts in different places or under different conditions. Follow a long workout with a short one, an intense session with a relaxed one, or high speed with easy distance. If your workouts become dull, do something different!

Warm-up and cool-down—You should always warm up before strenuous activity in order to increase your body temperature; increase your respiration and heart rate; and minimize your risk of muscle, tendon, and ligament strain.

Cooling down properly helps you avoid cramping and soreness, lowers your body temperature, and removes excess norepinephrine (too much left in your system can cause irregular heartbeats). In addition, cooling down with light activity and stretching will continue the pumping action of muscles on your veins, which will help your circulation remove metabolic wastes.

Long-term training—If you practice patience and allow your body systems to adapt comfortably to gradual overload, you will enjoy impressive improvements in performance—in due time. You cannot approach high-level performance capability in a day, a week, or a month. It takes years, but it pays off, because long-term training allows you to grow and develop, progress gradually, acquire skills, learn strategies, and gain a fuller understanding of your chosen sport.

Reversibility—The adaptations you coax from your body over months of hard training are mostly reversible. Inactivity will lead to loss of fitness and atrophy of your muscles. You can steer clear of this fate by persisting in a year-round program and alternating periods of hard work with periods of relative rest and variety.

Moderation—Too much of anything can be bad for you. So, sure, dedicate yourself to training faithfully, but temper your commitment with judgment and moderation. Train too hard, too fast, or too long and your body will deteriorate. Even elite athletes vary their training by mixing in easy days between hard sessions, and it's okay—indeed, crucial—for you to do the same.

Potential—Like everyone, you have a potential maximal level of performance. Most of us never get close to realizing this potential, but that's okay. In fact, it means that your best potential performances are still ahead of you! If you engage in regular physical activity, you will achieve more and more of your potential and improve the quality of your daily living.

Fallacies

You may come across other so-called facts about training, but you should be aware that some of them are actually fallacies or misconceptions. These oft-quoted statements are not true and have no basis in medical or scientific research.

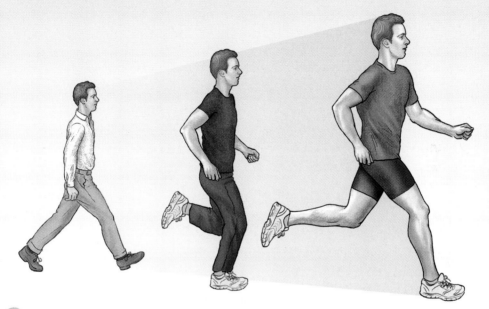

Train gradually, and you will soon get results without pain.

FALLACY 1 ➤ No Pain, No Gain

Although serious training is often difficult and sometimes unpleasant, it shouldn't actually hurt. Here is an important distinction: Pain is not a natural consequence of exercise or training; it signals a problem that you need to address. In fact, well-prepared athletes sometimes perform in a state of euphoria, free of pain and oblivious to discomfort. Think about it: You've probably seen the end of a long-distance race where the winner finishes full of life even though the rest of the field appears wasted. This is made possible by the fact that when you exercise, your body produces natural opiates (endorphins) that can mask discomfort of the effort. But if you suffer real pain while training, back off. And if the pain persists, get it evaluated.

All of this notwithstanding, discomfort can accompany difficult training such as heavy lifting, intense interval training, and long-distance

No Discomfort, No Excellence

work. This discomfort (as distinct from pain) results naturally from the lactic acid that accompanies the anaerobic effort of lifting or doing intense intervals—and of the muscle fatigue, microscopic muscle damage, and soreness that come with long-distance training. Thus, whereas I reject the "no pain, no gain" mantra, I accept the following statement: No discomfort, no excellence. Overload is necessary for adaptation, and it sometimes requires you to work at your limit of strength, intensity, or endurance, which certainly can be uncomfortable. But if your exercise results in outright pain, it is probably excessive.

FALLACY 2 ➤ You Must Break Down Muscle to Improve

Neither pain nor injury is a normal result of training—whether for muscular endurance or for strength—and you can avoid both of these outcomes. Weightlifters can traumatize their muscles by using excessive weight or doing excessive repetitions, but such trauma is not a necessary stage in the development of strength. Similarly, some people who train and compete vigorously experience microtrauma in their muscles, but this too is an unnecessary (and undesirable!) outcome of training. Some runners, for example, experience microtrauma at the end of a marathon that includes long downhill stretches requiring eccentric muscular contractions (i.e., contractions of a lengthening muscle). Such contractions are a major cause of muscle soreness, which is associated with muscle trauma, reduced force output, and a protracted recovery period (4 to 6 weeks). Thus, "breaking down" muscle does not help you train. It brings your training to a standstill.

FALLACY 3 ➤ Go for the Burn

This mantra is often heard among bodybuilders who do numerous repetitions and sets to build, shape, and define their muscles. They are probably referring to the sensation felt when the level of lactic acid increases in a muscle. This sensation is not dangerous, but it is not necessary, and you need not seek it out as part of a strength program to improve your fitness and health.

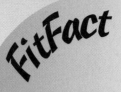

FALLACY 4 ➤ Lactic Acid Causes Muscle Soreness

This fallacy has been around for decades but has no basis in fact. Lactic acid may be produced when you perform contractions that lead to soreness, but lactic acid does not cause the soreness. It is, in fact, cleared from your muscles and blood within an hour after you finish exercising. Thus, it is long gone by the time you begin to experience soreness, which appears 24 hours after exercise. So what does cause soreness? It is probably related to microtrauma in muscle and connective tissue, and resultant swelling, when you engage in a new kind of exertion or exercise after a long layoff. Once you recover, you will be less prone to soreness when you do the activity again.

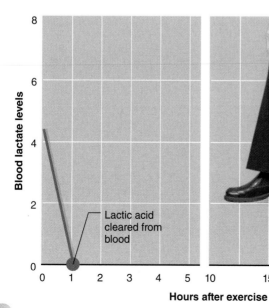

Lactic acid is long gone by the time you experience muscle soreness.

FALLACY 5 ➤ Muscle Turns to Fat (or Vice Versa)

Many people believe that if they stop exercising, their muscle will turn to fat. This is simply not true; neither muscle nor fat will turn into the other. Both are highly specialized kinds of tissue that play specific roles in your body. Muscles consist of spaghetti-like fibers that contain contractile proteins designed to exert force. Fat cells are round receptacles designed to store fat. The reason muscle grows or gets smaller is that training increases the size of muscle fibers (hypertrophy), whereas detraining reduces the size of these fibers (atrophy). Fat cells, in contrast, grow in size as they store more fat due to excess caloric consumption. If, on the other hand, you use more calories than you take in, fat cells shrink. But in no case do your long, thin muscle fibers change into spherical blobs of fat, or vice versa.

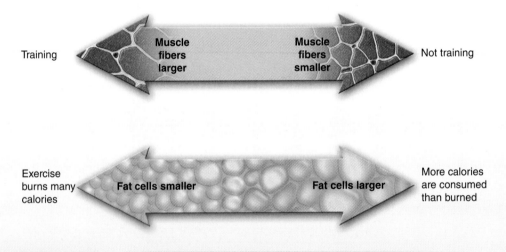

FALLACY 6 ➤ I Ran Out of Wind

If you run too fast for your level of training, you may feel as if you have run out of wind. This sensation comes from your lungs and is one example of the discomfort that can accompany vigorous exertion. The cause, however, is less likely a lack of oxygen or air and more likely an *excess* of carbon dioxide, which is produced when your body metabolizes carbohydrate. Thus, vigorous effort can lead to high levels of carbon dioxide, which can in turn create distress signals in your lungs. In this case, your respiratory system decides that it is more important to rid your body of excess CO_2 than to bring in more O_2. Excess CO_2 is a signal that you are working above your level of training—that you have exceeded the level of exertion you can sustain. If you ignore this sensation, you will become exhausted, but if you become familiar with it, you can use the sensation to regulate your exercise training.

FALLACY 7 ➤ If Seen on TV, It Must Be True

You've seen them—those 30-minute sales pitches for fitness equipment or exercise systems. Develop your abs, build your six-pack, exercise every muscle, whatever. The spokesperson promises quick results from little time or effort and may tout a money-back "guarantee." You almost never see the claims supported by research results gathered by an independent lab. Instead, you hear celebrity endorsements, often given by a beautiful actress or model or a well-known athlete. They suggest that the fitness program leads to impressive results far faster than old-fashioned ways of exercising. But they provide no evidence—just unverified testimonials. You should know that the equipment will soon clutter your garage, basement, or attic; that you'll need a lawyer to get your money back; and that there will be a new exercise miracle coming to your TV screen in just a few months. Just remember the old axiom: If it sounds too good to be true, it probably is.

beautiful body

Theories Require Proof

Some areas of exercise and training could use additional evidence to support their claims and justify any additional cost.

Q: Is Pilates more effective than other forms of stretching and strengthening exercises?

A: While Pilates is effective in developing flexibility and strength, so are other forms of exercise. Remember the principle of specificity: Pilates might help with alignment of your spine and strengthen your deep torso muscles, but targeted exercises may do more to help you meet your goals.

Q: Does balance training or tai chi improve your balance more than tennis or golf does?

A: While tai chi does improve balance, there is little evidence that it does so more than other forms of activity.

Q: Does static or dynamic stretching reduce the risk of injury?

A: More studies are needed to verify the effect of stretching on the risk of injury. However, stretching does reduce discomfort and may reduce the likelihood of muscle tightness and muscle pulls.

Q: Does yoga build strength as effectively as weightlifting does?

A: It is unlikely that yoga can build strength as effectively as a weightlifting program can.

Q: Does massage provide greater benefits than you get from active recovery and stretching?

A: Massage is quite popular, especially among world-class athletes who engage in strenuous and prolonged training. Massage feels good and it aids relaxation. Use it if you like, but remember, active recovery and rest allow recovery from most forms of exertion.

Keys to Fitness Facts and Fallacies

➤ Theories require experimental verification.

➤ Experimental studies validate training methods and techniques.

➤ If you try to rush your training, you risk illness, injury, or both.

➤ The type of training you undertake should relate to your desired results.

➤ Cross-training is a way to avoid overuse injuries.

➤ TV infomercials are based on endorsements, not carefully controlled studies.

What's Next?...

Now that you know the truth about common exercise facts and fallacies, move on to chapter 11 to learn how to remain active in your older years.

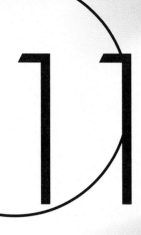

11

Vitality and Longevity

Add Life to Your Years

There are shortcuts to happiness,
and dancing is one of them.

~ Vicki Baum

Sophie

is an indefatigable 60-year-old grandmother.

She confronts life with boundless enthusiasm and handles a hectic schedule with charm and grace. Along with her regular half-time job, she teaches French, cooking, and music to pay the bills. Then it's off to rehearsal for one of two choral groups or for the church choir. In addition, at any one time Sophie might be planning and rehearsing for a solo recital, a jazz gig, or a role in a community theater production.

Where does she get all that energy?

Sophie

In her "spare time," she is a photographer who participates in exhibitions. And of course she is deeply involved in politics, local issues, and the peace movement. Sophie does all these things but does not engage in a fitness program. How does she pull it off? How does she juggle these involvements and still find time for family and friends? Where does she get all that *energy*? She dances! She dances with verve, ardor, and enthusiasm at local clubs and social events. She loves rock, Latin, salsa, and African rhythms. She does the tango and goes contra dancing. She even does country and swing. When possible, she walks or bikes around town, and she is trying to find time for skiing and hiking. She lives life to the fullest—and so can you.

Getting Older

The prevailing view of aging is a none-too-happy one. It offers a life of limits and ailments in which you are doomed to a vicious cycle of frailty and loss of function. You need not, however, allow this tragic tale to become *your* story. If you adopt an active and healthy lifestyle, you can write and perform from a different script—one that features a long and satisfying life. The decision is yours.

Life expectancies in the United States, which have risen throughout the past century, currently range from 78 to 79 for women and 73 to 74 for men. Even so, certain realities are inescapable: As your best reproductive years pass, the direct evolutionary advantage of your individual existence fades, and at some point most of your tissues and organs begin to age. Granted, you may remain important as a parent, at least until your child reaches young adulthood, and you may eventually be useful as a grandparent who passes on wisdom and helps out as needed. But once you reach your 70s, there is generally little *biological* justification for your life to continue.

Your age, however, does not tell your whole story. In fact, age alone reveals little about your fitness, health, appearance, or ability to perform. Of course, aging eventually leads to death for everyone, but it does so at different rates for different people, and the difference depends not only on heredity but also on decisions you make about how to age.

How do you want to age?

Life Span

As infant mortality and infectious disease have declined, human life expectancy has generally gone up. But the attainable life span—that is, the age attainable in a life that is free of serious illness and accident—has changed little over the past 200 years. Thus, we are not so much living longer but more effectively avoiding premature death. Research points to a current attainable life span of about 85 years in the United States; more specifically, about two-thirds of the population has the potential to live between 81 and 89 years, and nearly all people (95 percent) who die of natural causes live somewhere between 77 and 93 years.

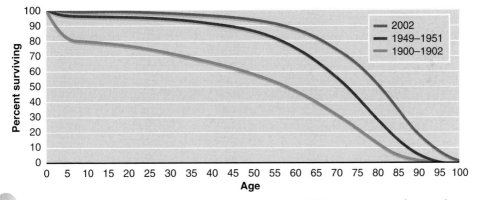

Percent surviving by age: Death-registration States, 1900 to 1902, and United States, 1949 to 1951 and 2002. With good health habits, more people are able to postpone chronic debilitating illness, remaining vigorous until the last years or months of life.

Reprinted from National Center for Health Statistics, 2004, p. 5.

As we have reduced and postponed the incidence of chronic illness, we have extended the duration of adult vigor. As a result, many people have the potential to remain physically, emotionally, and intellectually vigorous until shortly before the close of life. You make decisions every day that affect aspects of your health that become problematic with age, such as

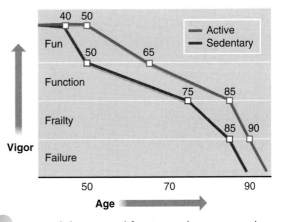

Vigor and the active life. Active living extends the period of fun and function and shortens the time of frailty and failure.

Reprinted by permission from Sharkey and Gaskill, 2007, p. 349.

heart and lung function, bone density, blood pressure, and cholesterol. Thus, you have a choice. If you decide to age rapidly, you are destined to become a burden to your family, to the health care system, and to community support systems. But if you choose to live an active, healthy life, you are likely to extend your vigorous years. Activity can add years to your life—and life to your years!

Leading an active life can increase your longevity. The least-fit people are much more likely to die from any cause than are those who are moderately or highly fit.

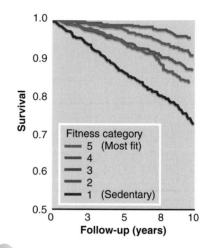

Death from any cause across various levels of fitness in healthy individuals.

Adapted by permission from Mandic, Myers, Oliveira, Abella, and Froelicher, 2009.

As seen in the graph to the right, when people were categorized into five levels of fitness, with 1 representing the least fit and 5 representing the most fit, the biggest difference in mortality was between those who were least fit (category 1) and those who were just one level fitter (category 2). But there were still gains in the higher levels of fitness, and people who were the least fit were *four times* more likely to die of anything, including cardiovascular events, than were the fittest people (Mandic et al. 2009). What's the bottom line? If you're not active at all right now, you can make a difference in your chances of living longer simply by adding a little activity. And the more active you are, the longer you are likely to live.

Some have lamented the fact that any years you add to your life will come at the end. Some have also suggested that whatever years you add are cancelled out by the time you spend exercising in order to get them. Let's look at the facts and think this through. One study found that activity was associated with an increase in life expectancy of 1 to more than 2 years (Paffenbarger et al. 1986). Let's assume that you spend 14,610 hours in exercise (1 hour every day for 40 years). That works out to 609 days, or 1.67 years, which is less than the 2 or more years you're likely to earn. Add to that the fact that you will enjoy the time you spend in exercise, recreation, and sport, and it's a pretty simple decision. Would you like to extend your years of fun and function—that is, the prime of your life?

FitFact

In most cases, you can extend your vigorous years by living an active, healthy lifestyle.

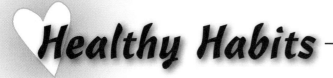Healthy Habits

Researchers have studied the relationship of health to various behaviors and habits. Health and longevity are associated with the following:

- Adequate sleep (7 to 8 hours per night)
- A good breakfast
- Regular meals (avoid snacks)
- Weight control
- Not smoking
- Little or no alcohol consumption (only one to two drinks per day)
- Regular exercise

The Human Population Laboratory concluded that men could add 11 years to their lives and women could add 7 years just by following six of these habits (Breslow and Enstrom 1980). So examine the list to see how it compares with your current lifestyle, and then decide whether any changes are in order.

Age and Performance

Your chronological age (how long you've lived) is less important than your physiological age (how well your body functions). Chronological age is, in fact, a poor predictor of your health and your performance in work or sport. Both health and performance are a function of your habits, your heredity, your environment, and any previous illness you've experienced. In other words, they are determined by your physiological age.

The best measure of your physiological age is probably your aerobic fitness, which involves the health and capacity of your respiratory, circulatory, and muscular systems. In addition, considerable research shows that when you improve your aerobic fitness, you reduce your risk of heart disease and cancer. As a result, it is possible for a 55-year-old to enjoy the health and performance of the average 25- to 30-year-old. Tell that to an employer who engages in age discrimination!

Add LIFE to your years, not just years to your life.

Longevity

If you're looking to live longer, beyond normal life expectancy, your approach to life is crucial. Regardless of occasional stories about centenarians who attribute their longevity to something like whiskey or fried eggs, purposeful observation of healthy persons who are 75 or older yields real insight into the traits and habits associated with long-term survival.

The following characteristics are associated with longevity:

➤ **Moderation.** Moderation is a good approach to all aspects of life, including diet, pleasure, work, and physical activity. Whether you are talking about a footrace or the human race, long-term success depends on pacing.

➤ **Flexibility.** Psychological flexibility involves the ability to bend but not break, to avoid rigid habits, and to accept change.

➤ **Challenges.** Don't let your life become too easy. Instead, accept challenges—and, if necessary, create them. At the same time, know when to say when. If a challenge becomes too great, acknowledge that fact and find an alternative.

➤ **Health habits.** Long-term survival is characterized by a relaxed attitude toward health. Elderly "survivors" are relatively unconcerned about their health. They tend to enjoy a wide variety of foods, are moderate in their use of alcohol, and may even smoke once in a while. They are living proof of the value of a moderate, balanced approach to a healthy lifestyle.

➤ **Relationships.** Older citizens value people. They tend to enjoy their marriages and actively maintain close contact with family and friends.

➤ **Outlook.** Healthy elders take a positive view of life. They realize that long life means growing old, and they acknowledge the effects of advancing age. This acceptance enables them to plan for and actively enjoy each phase of life.

➤ **Active life.** Those who age successfully get involved in various daily routines that require activity. They create ways to be socially and physically active, and their eager involvement in daily chores provides them with purpose, rhythm, and activity.

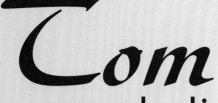

Tom

was rendered immovable by a series of life events. First, he underwent knee replacement surgery, and soon afterward he suffered a much more serious blow: His wife was diagnosed with cancer, and she soon passed away. Tom descended into a lonely depression. Friends and family members did what they could, and in time their encouragement and that of his two big dogs drew him out of the house. For the next 2 years, Tom's walks with his dogs and his interactions with family and friends largely defined the scope of his life. Then, as he approached his 70th birthday, an old friend told him about a woman, Gail, whom he might want to meet. She was a widow who lived 2,000 miles away, and after their first phone conversation turned out to be successful, it was quickly followed by many more. Eventually, Tom invited Gail for a visit, and it went well, but he realized that he would have to get in better shape in order to travel and keep up with his active new friend. He started taking 30-minute walks and, in due time, extended some of them to an hour. He also began working with light weights and bicycling a little. Now he travels and hikes with Gail throughout the country. They are making plans for a trip to Ireland, and perhaps more.

Living an active life can benefit you in a number of ways:

➤ **Health.** Both physical and mental health are enhanced by regular activity.

➤ **Mobility.** The combination of regular aerobic activity and resistance exercise enables you to retain or restore mobility—and your capacity for living freely and independently.

➤ **Economy.** Walk, jog, or ride a bike, and you'll save money. Cross-country skis are not only cheaper than a snowmobile, but they're also better for you!

➤ **Ecology.** Living actively and emphasizing muscle-powered sport and recreation helps conserve the planet's limited energy supply. If you are physically active, you will step more lightly on the earth than your sedentary peers who are inclined toward energy-consuming recreational vehicles and leaf blowers.

➤ **Adaptability.** Active individuals are better able to adapt to change—whether in life, the economy, or the environment.

➤ **Survival.** Seniors are survivors who have accumulated wisdom that is of great value to younger generations. Long-term research data indicate that, as it generally is in nature, so it is with the human race: The *fittest* survive.

Active individuals fully inhabit the present moment. They take risks, engage in life, and enjoy the ride. They don't waste the moment on moods or immobilizing worry. They avoid people who depress them, and when they do feel moody or depressed, they *do* something. Mood and the chemistry of behavior are complexly related, and physical activity can have a direct effect on both. Subtle changes in brain chemistry and hormone levels can lead to—or be caused by—depression, worry, guilt, and anger. Physical activity reduces depression, anxiety, and one's reaction to stress while it improves one's mood. It can also divert your attention,

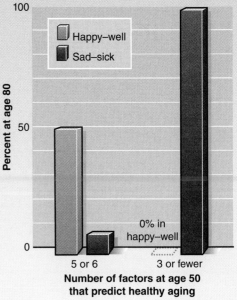

At age 50, if you have five or more of the factors found to predict successful aging, you are much more likely to be "happy–well" as opposed to "sad–sick" at age 80.

provide enjoyment, and foster a sense of self-satisfaction that minimizes or even eliminates self-defeating behavior. As an active older adult you might take charge in these ways:

➤ You are free to think and act as you desire. You are not bound by circumstances, astrological signs, biorhythms, behavioral traits, genetics, or deep-seated psychological problems.

➤ You can create the life you desire. Don't fall back on excuses such as "I haven't got the time," "I'll start next week (or month or year)," or "I'm too busy right now, but when the kids are a little older . . ."

➤ Finally, consider the "happy–well" group described in a longitudinal study by Vaillant (2001). Membership in the most successful group at age 80 was predicted by six factors measured at age 50: a stable marriage, a mature and adaptive approach to life, avoidance of smoking, little alcohol consumption, regular exercise, and maintenance of normal weight.

Stages of Life

Physical activity should be spontaneous and enjoyable, and excessive planning can lead to the drudgery that characterizes too many fitness programs. At the same time, a well-conceived plan can facilitate the flow of your life as one season melts into another. Why not give your physical life the same level of attention you give to work, finances, education, and travel?

It is not overreaching to say that each of us is engaged in a lifelong search for meaning. Along the way, our lives are characterized by an ebb and flow of purpose and confidence. Periods of doubt are followed by times of satisfaction, and our goals and interests shift as the stages of life unfold.

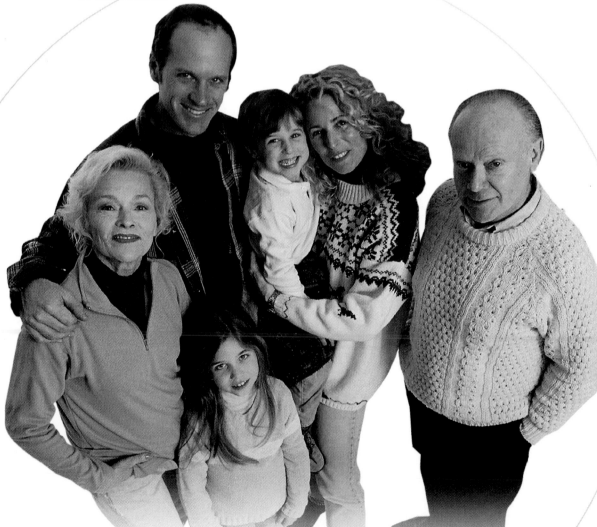

"Every age has its pleasures, its style of wit, and its own ways."

~Nicolas Boileau-Despréaux

STAGES OF LIFE

YOUNG ADULT

This stage generally requires cutting (or at least loosening) ties, getting educated, establishing a career, finding a mate, and perhaps starting a family. Thus, it is common to see success at this stage of life defined in educational and material terms.

ADULT

If he or she avoids divorce and major career changes, a 30-something adult might just be able, if the idea appeals, to purchase a home and put down some roots. That goal is often threatened by uncertainties, however, either in the workplace or the economy. This period may also find a person in the midst of what we call midlife crisis—a sense that time keeps on ticking and the opportunity to reach long-held goals may be slipping away. Between the ages of 45 and 55 years, however—the period sometimes called middle age—people often begin to accept themselves and their lives. They may redefine their goals for success and quality of life, and they may emerge from this process feeling refreshed. Indeed, if we are willing to let go of established roles and definitions, we may gain a renewed sense of purpose and thus enter the best time of life so far (Sheehy 1976).

STAGES OF LIFE

SENIOR

The senior stage, sometimes referred to as the golden years, may be in some ways the best of all. This stage may provide, at long last, the time and resources to fulfill personal goals. And even if resources are limited, seniors can experience deep satisfaction if their goals are qualitative rather than quantitative.

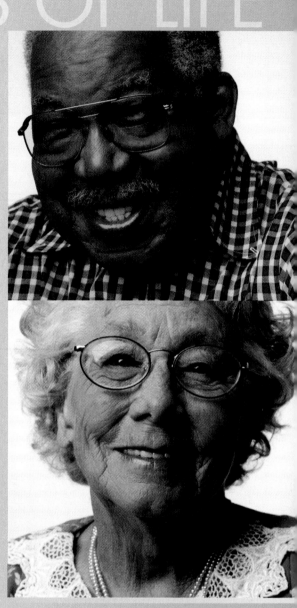

ELDER

Sometime after the age of 80, many folks say they begin to slow down—but not stop. Artists and musicians often continue to create and perform during this period. In spite of crippling rheumatoid arthritis, for example, my independent mother continued to play the piano in musical programs until shortly before her death at the age of 84. Gardening and swimming helped her maintain the physical vitality she needed in order to pursue her passion for music.

Some activities (American football comes to mind) should be attempted only by the young, whereas others are perfectly suited for adults, seniors, and even elders. Activities such as fishing, sailing, and golf, for example, can be enjoyed at any stage of life. Indeed, if you relax, you'll find that there is time for everything you really want to do. If you are still younger at this point, take some time to think about activities that you might want to take up in the future, when you have the time to enjoy them. As your age advances, you'll find new challenges and new adventures.

You may temporarily put aside favorite activities, but you'll never forget well-learned skills. If you enjoy engaging in competition, you'll find that it becomes more difficult as you approach the top of an age group; then, when you enter a new age group, it's like being a kid again! Sooner or later, most of us gravitate less toward competition and more toward cooperation—discovering, for example, the quiet beauty of sailing, the solitude of the wilderness, or the companionship afforded by golf and tennis. There is a season for everything, and if you keep active, you'll find time to enjoy all the seasons and stages of your life.

The Cost of Sloth

You know by now that physical inactivity exacts a price. It is responsible for major economic costs and is a major contributor to heart disease, diabetes, osteoporosis, and some forms of cancer. It may be responsible for as many as 407,000 deaths annually in the United States (Danaei et al. 2009). Little is being done, however, to reverse our slouch toward sloth and obesity. What *can* be done? Well, here are a few ideas:

Children and Adolescents

Restore school physical education programs.

Train and test for fitness.

Institute weight management programs.

Eliminate school-based fast food and soft drinks.

Restore after-school programs.

Initiate community-based and club programs.

Foster involvement in lifetime sports.

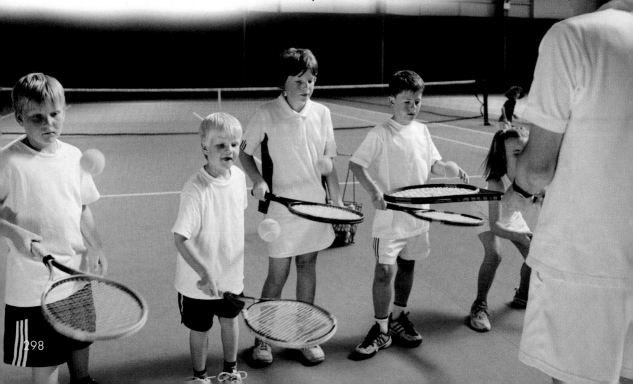

FitFact

The body doesn't wear out; it rusts out. Staying active can help you prevent an early decline.

Families

Discuss, plan, and engage in active recreation.

Emphasize nonmotorized (muscle-powered) activities.

Take active vacations.

Plan meaningful activities for every season.

Limit high-calorie desserts, snacks, and soft drinks.

Engage in active recreation.

Adults

Make time for physical activity and sport.

Give gifts that encourage activity.

Exercise outdoors when possible.

Use health and fitness clubs.

Participate in worksite employee health (wellness) programs.

Plan meaningful activities for every season.

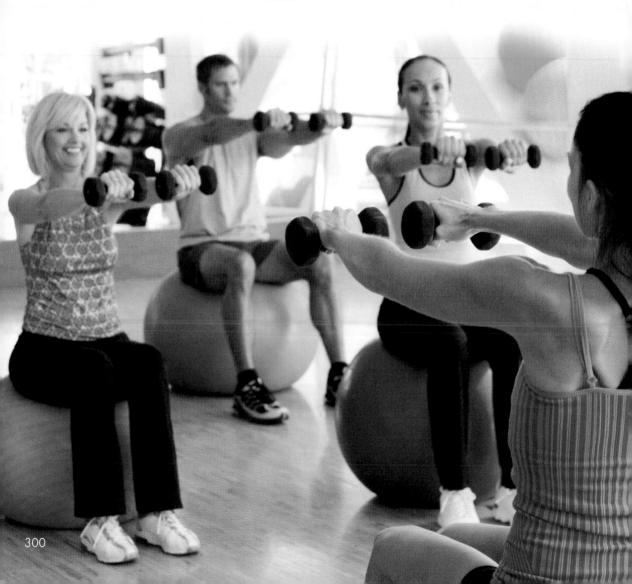

Seniors

Be active in every season.

Engage in aerobic and muscular fitness training.

Make use of community and health club resources.

Train for travel: Walk and weight train.

Participate with children and grandchildren.

Elders

Walk for physical and mental health.

Do muscular fitness training to maintain mobility.

Remain socially active.

socialize

Environment and Quality of Life

Become involved in local causes that improve your neighborhood and the quality of life it affords. Help maintain parks, open spaces, and the physical environment. Pursue construction of bike lanes, hiking trails, swimming pools, and skate parks. Since physical activity is associated with health, officials at all levels of government should consider the health implications of their actions. Encourage your local, state, and national legislators and agency administrators to consider how laws and regulations affect health and quality of life.

Just as land-use policies require environmental impact analyses prior to authorizing changes in land use, we should require a health impact analysis before approving any law or policy. Would this emphasis hurt the economy? To the contrary, healthy behaviors are usually good for the economy and the environment. For example, nonmotorized physical activity conserves fuel, doesn't pollute, and is easy on the environment and far less expensive for participants. A mountain bike is cheaper than an all-terrain vehicle; a canoe or kayak is much cheaper than a personal watercraft; and cross-country skis are far cheaper than a snowmobile.

Keys to Vitality and Longevity

➤ Be active almost every day.

➤ Select meaningful pursuits.

➤ Be sure to do muscular fitness training, including core training, as you age.

➤ Practice moderation in all aspects of life, including physical activity.

➤ Plan for and enjoy each phase of your life.

What's Next?...

It is up to you. What decisions will you make? What goals will you set? If you haven't done so already, now is the time to make a commitment to the active life—and to share that commitment with your family and friends. Start today by choosing one small way in which you will be active and enjoy the moment. Identify meaningful activities that fit each season of the year. In time, you will be able to expand your horizons as you experience the benefits of activity and fitness, and one day you will look back and see how your vigor has enhanced each stage of life. BEGIN TODAY—you will never regret the decision!

Appendix

Energy Expenditure Chart

	kg	54	64	73	82	91	100	109	118	127
Activities	**lb**	**120**	**140**	**160**	**180**	**200**	**220**	**240**	**260**	**280**

ESTIMATED CALORIES BURNED PER MINUTE OF ACTIVITY

Light

Activities	120	140	160	180	200	220	240	260	280
Child care (sitting or kneeling)	2.4	2.8	3.2	3.6	4.0	4.4	4.8	5.2	5.6
Cleaning, light (dusting; picking up; cleaning sink, tub, or toilet)	2.4	2.8	3.2	3.6	4.0	4.4	4.8	5.2	5.6
Cooking	1.9	2.2	2.6	2.9	3.2	3.5	3.8	4.1	4.4
Croquet	2.4	2.8	3.2	3.6	4.0	4.4	4.8	5.2	5.6
Fishing from boat	2.4	2.8	3.2	3.6	4.0	4.4	4.8	5.2	5.6
Fishing (ice)	1.9	2.2	2.6	2.9	3.2	3.5	3.8	4.1	4.4
Hand-sewing	1.9	2.2	2.6	2.9	3.2	3.5	3.8	4.1	4.4
Horseback riding at a walk	2.4	2.8	3.2	3.6	4.0	4.4	4.8	5.2	5.6
Ironing	2.2	2.6	2.9	3.3	3.7	4.0	4.4	4.7	5.1
Mowing lawn with riding mower	2.4	2.8	3.2	3.6	4.0	4.4	4.8	5.2	5.6
Playing catch	2.4	2.8	3.2	3.6	4.0	4.4	4.8	5.2	5.6
Playing pool	2.4	2.8	3.2	3.6	4.0	4.4	4.8	5.2	5.6
Shooting (pistol or trap)	2.4	2.8	3.2	3.6	4.0	4.4	4.8	5.2	5.6
Shopping	2.2	2.6	2.9	3.3	3.7	4.0	4.4	4.7	5.1
Sitting while playing cards, at sporting event, in meeting	1.4	1.7	1.9	2.2	2.4	2.6	2.9	3.1	3.3
Sitting while typing, writing	1.7	2.0	2.3	2.6	2.9	3.2	3.4	3.7	4.0
Sleeping	0.9	1.0	1.1	1.3	1.4	1.6	1.7	1.9	2.0
Standing	1.7	2.0	2.3	2.6	2.9	3.2	3.4	3.7	4.0
Stretching	2.4	2.8	3.2	3.6	4.0	4.4	4.8	5.2	5.6
Walking at 30 minutes per mile (1.6 km)	2.4	2.8	3.2	3.6	4.0	4.4	4.8	5.2	5.6
Washing dishes while standing	2.2	2.6	2.9	3.3	3.7	4.0	4.4	4.7	5.1
Watching TV while sitting or lying	1.0	1.1	1.3	1.4	1.6	1.8	1.9	2.1	2.2

Activities		ESTIMATED CALORIES BURNED PER MINUTE OF ACTIVITY								
	kg	54	64	73	82	91	100	109	118	127
	lb	120	140	160	180	200	220	240	260	280
Moderate										
Aerobic dance (low impact)		4.8	5.6	6.4	7.2	8.0	8.8	9.5	10.3	11.1
Archery		3.4	3.9	4.5	5.0	5.6	6.1	6.7	7.2	7.8
Badminton		4.3	5.0	5.7	6.5	7.2	7.9	8.6	9.3	10.0
Bicycling at 10 miles (16 km) per hour		3.9	4.5	5.1	5.7	6.4	7.0	7.6	8.3	8.9
Bowling		2.9	3.4	3.8	4.3	4.8	5.3	5.7	6.2	6.7
Canoeing		3.9	4.5	5.1	5.7	6.4	7.0	7.6	8.3	8.9
Carpentry, general		2.9	3.4	3.8	4.3	4.8	5.3	5.7	6.2	6.7
Carrying small children		2.9	3.4	3.8	4.3	4.8	5.3	5.7	6.2	6.7
Cleaning, heavy (mopping, vacuuming)		3.4	3.9	4.5	5.0	5.6	6.1	6.7	7.2	7.8
Dancing (line, polka, country)		4.3	5.0	5.7	6.5	7.2	7.9	8.6	9.3	10.0
Dancing (waltz, foxtrot, samba)		2.9	3.4	3.8	4.3	4.8	5.3	5.7	6.2	6.7
Fishing from bank		3.4	3.9	4.5	5.0	5.6	6.1	6.7	7.2	7.8
Frisbee with light effort		2.9	3.4	3.8	4.3	4.8	5.3	5.7	6.2	6.7
Golf with no cart		4.3	5.0	5.7	6.5	7.2	7.9	8.6	9.3	10.0
Kayaking		4.8	5.6	6.4	7.2	8.0	8.8	9.5	10.3	11.1
Laying sod		4.8	5.6	6.4	7.2	8.0	8.8	9.5	10.3	11.1
Marching band		3.9	4.5	5.1	5.7	6.4	7.0	7.6	8.3	8.9
Mowing lawn with power mower		4.3	5.0	5.7	6.5	7.2	7.9	8.6	9.3	10.0
Painting (exterior)		4.8	5.6	6.4	7.2	8.0	8.8	9.5	10.3	11.1
Painting (interior)		2.9	3.4	3.8	4.3	4.8	5.3	5.7	6.2	6.7
Raking lawn		3.9	4.5	5.1	5.7	6.4	7.0	7.6	8.3	8.9
Shuffleboard		2.9	3.4	3.8	4.3	4.8	5.3	5.7	6.2	6.7
Skateboarding		4.8	5.6	6.4	7.2	8.0	8.8	9.5	10.3	11.1
Snorkeling		4.8	5.6	6.4	7.2	8.0	8.8	9.5	10.3	11.1
Snowmobiling		3.4	3.9	4.5	5.0	5.6	6.1	6.7	7.2	7.8
Softball		4.8	5.6	6.4	7.2	8.0	8.8	9.5	10.3	11.1
Sweeping sidewalk		3.9	4.5	5.1	5.7	6.4	7.0	7.6	8.3	8.9

(continued)

(continued)

Activities	kg	54	64	73	82	91	100	109	118	127
ESTIMATED CALORIES BURNED PER MINUTE OF ACTIVITY	lb	120	140	160	180	200	220	240	260	280

Moderate *(continued)*

Activities	54 / 120	64 / 140	73 / 160	82 / 180	91 / 200	100 / 220	109 / 240	118 / 260	127 / 280
Swimming (treading water)	3.9	4.5	5.1	5.7	6.4	7.0	7.6	8.3	8.9
Table tennis	3.9	4.5	5.1	5.7	6.4	7.0	7.6	8.3	8.9
Tai chi	3.9	4.5	5.1	5.7	6.4	7.0	7.6	8.3	8.9
Trampoline	3.4	3.9	4.5	5.0	5.6	6.1	6.7	7.2	7.8
Trimming shrubs with manual clippers	4.3	5.0	5.7	6.5	7.2	7.9	8.6	9.3	10.0
Walking at 15 minutes per mile (1.6 km)	4.8	5.6	6.4	7.2	8.0	8.8	9.5	10.3	11.1
Walking at 20 minutes per mile	3.2	3.7	4.2	4.7	5.3	5.8	6.3	6.8	7.3
Washing and waxing a vehicle	2.9	3.4	3.8	4.3	4.8	5.3	5.7	6.2	6.7
Water aerobics	3.9	4.5	5.1	5.7	6.4	7.0	7.6	8.3	8.9
Weeding, digging in garden	4.3	5.0	5.7	6.5	7.2	7.9	8.6	9.3	10.0

Hard

Activities	54 / 120	64 / 140	73 / 160	82 / 180	91 / 200	100 / 220	109 / 240	118 / 260	127 / 280
Aerobic dance (high impact)	6.7	7.8	8.9	10.0	11.1	12.3	13.4	14.5	15.6
Carpentry (fence building, roofing)	5.8	6.7	7.7	8.6	9.6	10.5	11.4	12.4	13.3
Chopping wood	5.8	6.7	7.7	8.6	9.6	10.5	11.4	12.4	13.3
Circuit training	7.7	9.0	10.2	11.5	12.7	14.0	15.3	16.5	17.8
Fishing while wading in stream	5.8	6.7	7.7	8.6	9.6	10.5	11.4	12.4	13.3
Horseback riding at a trot	6.3	7.3	8.3	9.3	10.4	11.4	12.4	13.4	14.4
Marching	6.3	7.3	8.3	9.3	10.4	11.4	12.4	13.4	14.4
Moving furniture	5.8	6.7	7.7	8.6	9.6	10.5	11.4	12.4	13.3
Mowing lawn with hand mower	5.8	6.7	7.7	8.6	9.6	10.5	11.4	12.4	13.3
Race walking	6.3	7.3	8.3	9.3	10.4	11.4	12.4	13.4	14.4
Racquetball (casual)	6.7	7.8	8.9	10.0	11.1	12.3	13.4	14.5	15.6
Rowing with moderate effort	6.7	7.8	8.9	10.0	11.1	12.3	13.4	14.5	15.6
Sawing wood by hand	6.7	7.8	8.9	10.0	11.1	12.3	13.4	14.5	15.6
Shoveling (light to moderate)	6.3	7.3	8.3	9.3	10.4	11.4	12.4	13.4	14.4
Skating (roller or ice)	6.7	7.8	8.9	10.0	11.1	12.3	13.4	14.5	15.6
Ski machine	6.7	7.8	8.9	10.0	11.1	12.3	13.4	14.5	15.6
Skiing downhill with moderate effort	5.8	6.7	7.7	8.6	9.6	10.5	11.4	12.4	13.3
Skin diving	6.7	7.8	8.9	10.0	11.1	12.3	13.4	14.5	15.6
Swimming laps with light or moderate effort	6.7	7.8	8.9	10.0	11.1	12.3	13.4	14.5	15.6
Swimming (leisure)	5.8	6.7	7.7	8.6	9.6	10.5	11.4	12.4	13.3

	kg	54	64	73	82	91	100	109	118	127
ESTIMATED CALORIES BURNED PER MINUTE OF ACTIVITY										
Activities	lb	120	140	160	180	200	220	240	260	280

Hard *(continued)*

Activities	54/120	64/140	73/160	82/180	91/200	100/220	109/240	118/260	127/280
Tennis (doubles)	5.8	6.7	7.7	8.6	9.6	10.5	11.4	12.4	13.3
Walking with backpack	6.7	7.8	8.9	10.0	11.1	12.3	13.4	14.5	15.6
Weightlifting with vigorous effort	5.8	6.7	7.7	8.6	9.6	10.5	11.4	12.4	13.3

Very Hard

Activities	54/120	64/140	73/160	82/180	91/200	100/220	109/240	118/260	127/280
Basketball	7.7	9.0	10.2	11.5	12.7	14.0	15.3	16.5	17.8
Bicycling at 12 to 14 miles (19–23 km) per hour	7.7	9.0	10.2	11.5	12.7	14.0	15.3	16.5	17.8
Bicycling at 16 to 19 miles (26–31 km) per hour	11.6	13.4	15.3	17.2	19.1	21.0	22.9	24.8	26.7
Canoeing with vigorous effort	11.6	13.4	15.3	17.2	19.1	21.0	22.9	24.8	26.7
Cross-country skiing	8.7	10.1	11.5	12.9	14.3	15.8	17.2	18.6	20.0
Digging ditches	8.2	9.5	10.9	12.2	13.5	14.9	16.2	17.6	18.9
Football	7.7	9.0	10.2	11.5	12.7	14.0	15.3	16.5	17.8
Handball	11.6	13.4	15.3	17.2	19.1	21.0	22.9	24.8	26.7
Hockey (field or ice)	7.7	9.0	10.2	11.5	12.7	14.0	15.3	16.5	17.8
Horseback riding at a gallop	7.7	9.0	10.2	11.5	12.7	14.0	15.3	16.5	17.8
In-line skating	12.0	14.0	16.0	17.9	19.9	21.9	23.8	25.8	27.8
Martial arts (judo, karate, kickboxing)	9.6	11.2	12.8	14.4	15.9	17.5	19.1	20.7	22.2
Mountain biking	8.2	9.5	10.9	12.2	13.5	14.9	16.2	17.6	18.9
Racquetball (competitive)	9.6	11.2	12.8	14.4	15.9	17.5	19.1	20.7	22.2
Rowing with vigorous effort	11.6	13.4	15.3	17.2	19.1	21.0	22.9	24.8	26.7
Running at 8 minutes per mile (1.6 km)	12.0	14.0	16.0	17.9	19.9	21.9	23.8	25.8	27.8
Running at 10 minutes per mile	9.6	11.2	12.8	14.4	15.9	17.5	19.1	20.7	22.2
Skipping rope	7.7	9.0	10.2	11.5	12.7	14.0	15.3	16.5	17.8
Snowshoeing	10.6	12.3	14.1	15.8	17.5	19.3	21.0	22.7	24.4
Soccer	9.6	11.2	12.8	14.4	15.9	17.5	19.1	20.7	22.2
Stair stepper machine	8.7	10.1	11.5	12.9	14.3	15.8	17.2	18.6	20.0
Step aerobics with 6- to 8-inch (15–20 cm) step	8.2	9.5	10.9	12.2	13.5	14.9	16.2	17.6	18.9
Swimming with vigorous effort	10.6	12.3	14.1	15.8	17.5	19.3	21.0	22.7	24.4
Tennis (singles)	7.7	9.0	10.2	11.5	12.7	14.0	15.3	16.5	17.8
Volleyball	7.7	9.0	10.2	11.5	12.7	14.0	15.3	16.5	17.8
Walking at 12 minutes per mile (1.6 km)	7.7	9.0	10.2	11.5	12.7	14.0	15.3	16.5	17.8

Adapted by permission from Blair, Dunn, Marcus, Carpenter, and Jaret, 2001, pp. 179-182.

Bibliography

American College of Sports Medicine. 2005. *ACSM guidelines for exercise testing and prescription*. 6th ed. Baltimore: Lippincott Williams and Wilkins.

American Heart Association. *Risk factors and coronary heart disease*. www.americanheart.org/presenter.jhtml?identifier=4726.

Åstrand, P.O., and K. Rodahl. 1970. *Textbook of work physiology: Physiological bases of exercise*. 2nd ed. New York: McGraw-Hill.

Borg, G. 1973. Perceived exertion: A note on history and methods. *Medicine & Science in Sports & Exercise* 5:90-3.

Bouchard, C., M. Boulay, J. Simoneau, G. Lorrie, and L. Pierrise. 1988. Heritability and trainability of aerobic and anaerobic performance: An update. *Sports Medicine* 5:69-73.

Breslow, L., and J. Enstrom. 1980. Persistence of health habits and their relationship to mortality. *Preventive Medicine* 9:469-83.

Centers for Disease Control and Prevention. *National health and nutrition examination survey*. www.cdc.gov/nchs/nhanes.

Centers for Disease Control and Prevention. *Obesity and overweight*. www.cdc.gov/nchs/fastats/overwt.htm.

Danaei, G., E. Ding, D. Mozaffarian, B. Taylor, J. Rehm, C. Murray, and M. Ezzati. 2009. Preventable causes of death in the United States: Risk assessment of dietary, lifestyle, and metabolic risk factors. *PLoS Medicine* 6(4):e1000058.

Eichner, R. 1995. Contagious infections in competitive sports. *Sports Science Exchange* 8(3):1-4.

Fiatarone, M., E. O'Neill, N. Doyle Ryan, K. Clements, G. Solares, M. Nelson, S. Roberts, J. Kehayias, L. Lipsitz, and W. Evans. 1994. Exercise training and nutritional supplementation for physical frailty in very elderly people. *New England Journal of Medicine* 330:1769-75.

Frederick, E.C. 1973. *The running body*. Mountain View, CA: World Publications.

Fries, J., and L. Crapo. 1981. *Vitality and aging*. San Francisco: W.H. Freeman.

Holloszy, J.O. 1967. Biochemical adaptations in muscle: Effects of exercise on mitochondrial oxygen uptake and respiratory enzyme activity in skeletal muscle. *Journal of Biological Chemistry* 242:2278-82.

Institute of Medicine. 2002. *Dietary reference intakes for energy, carbohydrate, fiber, fat, fatty acids, cholesterol, protein, and amino acids*. books.nap.edu/openbook.php?record_id=104908page=880.

Keys, A., J. Brozek, A. Henschel, O. Mickelsen, and H. Taylor. 1950. *The biology of human starvation*. Volume I. Minneapolis: University of Minnesota Press.

Mandic, S., J. Myers, R. Oliveira, J. Abella, and V. Froelicher. 2009. Characterizing differences in mortality at the low end of the fitness spectrum. *Medicine & Science in Sports & Exercise* 41(8):1573-79.

Mehrotra, A., A. Zaslavsky, and J. Ayanian. 2007. Preventive health examinations and preventive gynecological examinations in the United States. *Archives of Internal Medicine* 167:1876-83.

Morgan, W.P. 2001. Prescription of physical activity: A paradigm shift. *Quest* 53:366-82.

Paffenbarger, R.S., R.T. Hyde, A.L. Wing, and C.C. Hsieh. 1986. Physical activity, all-cause mortality, and longevity of college alumni. *New England Journal of Medicine* 314:605-13.

Pate, R.R., M. Pratt, S.N. Blair, W.L. Haskell, C.A. Macera, C. Bouchard, D. Buchner, et al. 1995. Physical activity and public health: A recommendation from the Centers for Disease Control and Prevention and the American College of Sports Medicine. *JAMA* 273:402-7. wonder.cdc.gov/wonder/prevguid/p0000391/p0000391.asp.

President's Council on Physical Fitness and Sport. 1975. *An introduction to physical fitness.* Washington, D.C.: President's Council on Physical Fitness and Sport.

Sharkey, B.J., and P.O. Davis. 2008. *Hard work.* Champaign, IL: Human Kinetics.

Sharkey, B.J., and S.E. Gaskill. 2006. *Sport physiology for coaches.* Champaign, IL: Human Kinetics.

Sharkey, B.J., and S.E. Gaskill. 2007. *Fitness and health.* 6th ed. Champaign, IL: Human Kinetics.

Sheehy, G. 1976. *Passages: Predictable crises of adult life.* New York: Bantam.

Simoes, E., T. Byers, R. Coates, M. Serdula, A. Mokdad, and G. Heath. 1995. The association between leisure-time physical activity and dietary fat in American adults. *American Journal of Public Health* 85:240-4.

Siscovick, D., R. LaPorte, and J. Newman. 1985. The disease-specific benefits and risks of physical activity and exercise. *Public Health Reports* 100:180-8.

Thompson, P., B. Franklin, G. Balady, S. Blair, D. Corrado, M. Estes, J. Fulton, et al. 2007. Exercise and acute cardiovascular events: Placing the risks in perspective. *Medicine & Science in Sports & Exercise* 39:866-97.

U.S. Department of Health and Human Services. *2008 physical activity guidelines for Americans.* www.health.gov/paguidelines.

Vaillant, G. 2001. *Aging well.* New York: Little, Brown.

Index

Note: The italicized *f* and *t* following page numbers refer to figures and tables, respectively.

skiing, cross-country 60
skill 120-121
slow-twitch muscle fibers 100, 102, 104
special considerations, for exercise 251-253
specificity 27, 109-111, 117, 121, 135, 179, 267-268, 276
speed 115-116, 128*t*
spine stretch 158
spotter 133, 135
sprain, ankle 246
squat stretch 157
stability ball exercises 169-170
stability ball push-up 169
stages of life 294-297
stamina. *See* aerobic fitness
standing groin stretch 155
starter (walk–jog) program 68-77
static balance 116-117
static stretches. *See also specific stretches*
    injury risk and 277
    overview 140-142
status study 262-263
stop signs 243
strength
    decline in 98, 100
    defined 103-105
    goals 129-130
    improving 137
    leg 128*t*, 177-178, 180
    maintaining 138
    muscular fitness test for 128*t*
strength training. *See also specific exercises*
    guidelines 174, 183
    for hiking 132
    leg 128*t*, 177-178, 180
    muscles chosen for 131-132
    muscular fitness and 106-111, 111*t*
    muscular programs 174-182
    prescription 175
    upper-body 179
    yoga *v.* 113, 278
stretching. *See also* dynamic stretches; static stretches
    contract-and-relax 142, 157
    how-tos 144
    massage *v.* 279
    muscle pulls prevented with 247
supine leg curl 170
supplements 213, 216-218
surgery, for weight loss 225
swimming 60, 62, 69, 87

T
tai chi 277
tests 24-26, 70-71, 128*t*
training. *See also* aerobic fitness training; muscular fitness training
    balance 277
    defined 13
    effect 11
    flexibility 139-141, 145

    long-term 270
    principles 265-270
    specificity 27, 109-111, 117, 121, 135, 179, 267-268
    tips 89-93
trans-fatty acids 203-204
transfer RNA (tRNA) 107-108
travel 254
triceps dip 179
triglycerides 202-204
tRNA. *See* transfer RNA
trunk lift 164
trunk muscles, core training for 164-165
trunk stretch 154
TV advertisements 275
2008 Physical Activity Guidelines for Americans 9, 236

U
upper-body strength training 179
upper-hamstring and hip stretch 157
upper-shoulder stretch 154

V
variation 185, 269
vascular problems 5
vegetarianism 207
vertical jump 128*t*
vitality 282-283, 303
vitamins 212-217

W
walking
    activity selection 57-58, 62
    dynamic walking exercises 161
    programs 68-77
    test 70
walking knee lift 160
walk–jog program 68-77
walk–jog test 71
warm-up 113, 128, 140, 144, 269
warning signs 242-243
water-soluble vitamins 213
weight control
    dieting and 223-224
    energy expenditure and 222-223
    energy intake and 220-221
    keys to 231
    overview 219
    physical activity and 223-227
    practical weight loss program for 228-231
    surgery for 225
weight training program 188. *See also* muscular fitness training
white walk–jog program 74-75
wind, running out of 274
women 251-252
work 254

Y
yield signs 243
yoga 113, 278
young adult stage 295

About the Author

Brian Sharkey, PhD,

is a leading fitness researcher, educator, and author. Sharkey has more than 45 years of experience in exercise, sport, and work physiology. He is professor emeritus at the University of Montana, where he served as director of the Human Performance Laboratory and remains associated with the university and lab. He currently serves as a consultant with several federal agencies in the areas of fitness, health, and work capacity, especially of wildland firefighters. He has won several awards for his work, including the 2009 International 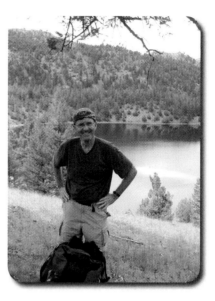 Association of Wildland Fire's Wildland Fire Safety Award for his contributions to wildland firefighter safety and health.

Sharkey authored or contributed to over a dozen books on exercise, sport, and work physiology and fitness and numerous research papers. He is past president of the American College of Sports Medicine and served on the NCAA committee on competitive safeguards and medical aspects of sports, where he chaired the Sports Science and Safety subcommittee, which uses research to improve the safety of intercollegiate athletics. He also coordinated the United States ski team Nordic Sports Medicine Council.

In his leisure time, Brian enjoys cross-country and alpine skiing, road and mountain biking, running and hiking in the hills and valleys, and paddling the rivers and lakes of Montana. He lives with his wife, Ann, close to his daughter, son, and grandchildren in Missoula, Montana.